HEARTS ON THE MEND

by Floriana Hall

To Karen:
Enjoy each day!
Love + Blessings,
Floriana Hall
12/31/06

PublishAmerica
Baltimore

First printing

At the specific preference of the author, PublishAmerica allowed this work to remain exactly as the author intended, verbatim, without editorial input.

ISBN: 1-4241-2038-1
PUBLISHED BY PUBLISHAMERICA, LLLP
www.publishamerica.com
Baltimore

Printed in the United States of America

This book is dedicated to all doctors and heart surgeons, heart patients, and scientists who discover newer and better methods every day to help prevent heart disease.

Acknowledgements

I want to thank all of the heart patients who shared their stories with me: Patricia Albanese, Jerry Bean, the late Joann Schindler, Doris Irvine, Judy Saunders, Daniel and Julie Lance, Gloria Pimentel, Ed and Peg Mitchell, a physician who chose to remain anonymous, and last, but not least, my brother Frank.

PROLOGUE

In 1929, Werner Forrsman, a surgical resident at a small country hospital in Germany, discovered the use of a catheter to detect heart disease. Soon others used catheters to discover how the heart pumps and how disease affects its functions. In 1956, Werner Forrsman, Dickinson Richards and Andre Cournand shared a Nobel Prize for their efforts in studying heart function using catheters.

Today, two thirds of people survive their heart attacks because Dr. Marcus DeWood of Spokane, Washington, began to use angiography to look at blockages of victims of heart attacks. In 1980, Dr. DeWood published articles proving that most heart attacks were caused by clots blocking an artery. If clot-busting medicine breaks up the clot quickly, the survival rate is higher.

Andreas Gruntzig performed the first angioplasty in 1977 to break up clots in narrow and hardened arteries. Stents are now used to hold the artery open.

Many hospitals now have "cath labs" where they can immediately do angioplasty when a heart attack patient arrives. If they aren't equipped with these labs, they administer clot busters.

Today, two thirds of people survive heart attacks, actually more men than women. Heart attacks are the leading cause of death for women age thirty-five and older.

Prevention, consisting of diet, exercise, not smoking or quitting smoking and taking cholesterol lowering drugs, if needed, is still important.

There have been and will be new methods discovered in the future, perhaps with less invasive surgery, perhaps even with robots. Only time will tell.

This book is written with the intent of helping doctors, surgeons, and the general public understand what a patient with heart disease experiences before and after surgery, and to help all people understand that it is necessary to be checked, using various methods, for heart disease.

The stories included in this book are all true, but the opinions expressed in some of them are not necessarily endorsed by the author.

FLORIANA HALL'S STORY

In the last two decades, medical science has advanced to such a degree that double, triple, or quadruple bypass heart surgery has become almost commonplace. There are separate heart groups and separate cardiac floors in many or most hospitals.

In my particular case, I am recovering from quadruple heart bypass surgery which was performed at City Hospital, Akron, Ohio, on September 4, 2003. City Hospital is part of Summa Health System which involves three hospitals in Akron; City, Akron General Medical Center, St. Thomas Hospital, and Cuyahoga Falls General Hospital in Cuyahoga Falls, Ohio, a suburb of Akron.

My story is unusual because I had no typical symptoms of heart trouble beforehand, such as chest pains, shortness of breath or heart palpitations. I attributed any tiredness I experienced to my age. I will be seventy-six years old (or young, depending on how you look at it) on October 2, 2003.

Each time I visited my knowledgeable young doctor, Dr. Lisa Altuglu, she listened to my heart and my carotid arteries and said, "Everything is fine," and I went on my merry way.

Since I am an author and poet, with seven books to my credit, I feel compelled to write this story in order to help others realize that it is necessary to have an EKG and/or stress test even when one has no symptoms of heart disease. My priorities in life are God, family, friends, country and helping people. Perhaps this book will save others' lives.

My wonderful mother passed away August 16, 1965, from a coronary occlusion at the young age of fifty-nine. She was working, healthy, happy and was even taking swimming lessons at the time. My two siblings and I could not understand what caused her death since she had no symptoms, so we had an autopsy performed and discovered that all of her arteries were blocked with plaque which had built up throughout her years of eating eggs and liver and onions which she so enjoyed. Of course, the genetic factor was present in which one's liver overproduces cholesterol. In those days, no one knew about the effects of cholesterol.

Perhaps, because of my mother's untimely death, I should have been on the lookout for some signs, but I was enjoying my active life. My former doctor had ruled out the stress test because it sometimes produced false-positive results. I had never had a stress test, even though, at the age of 54, I found out that my cholesterol was nearly 500 and my triglycerides were almost 1000. My doctor told me to lose weight, so I lost forty-five pounds. However, my cholesterol only dropped ten points from 497 down to 487. Losing weight was not the answer because it did not make much difference in my cholesterol count. It was determined that my liver was overproducing cholesterol, the same genetic problem as my mother.

Since that time, I have watched my diet closely, eating mostly no fat or low fat foods. Of course, being a chocoholic does not help, but I always limited myself, and I still do, to one candy bar a week, or one small piece of chocolate a day. I eat nonfat chocolate pudding several times a month to satisfy my craving for chocolate. If I ever cheat, it has to be a chocolate treat.

My doctor prescribed Lovastatin, or Mevacor, which had been the only cholesterol lowering medication my sensitive digestive system could tolerate.

Due to one gall bladder attack, my gallbladder and stones were removed thirteen years ago. That seemed to be the source of my stomach and digestive distress which I have experienced since. Maybe God was trying to tell me something, for I could not digest foods such as peanuts, peanut butter, popcorn, spaghetti sauce, fatty meats, and chocolate, all of which I had no problem eating before the surgery. I still have the same digestive problems at the present time.

Many people my age have undergone numerous operations, but, outside of having five children, I had had only one earlier surgery, a local tonsillectomy at the age of nineteen. I remember taking the bus home the next day and being enticed by the aroma of a fried hamburger with onions. I ate this hamburger against my mother's advice. It resulted in a month of bleeding which I will never forget. Even my friends from high school remember that incident like it was yesterday. The summer of my nineteenth year, I also had constant nose bleeds, and realized that I must be a person who bleeds easily, although I'm not a hemophiliac.

What does all this have to do with my story? Actually, a lot, but at that time it seemed insignificant. Twenty-five years after the tonsillectomy, when I had four wisdom teeth extracted, my gums bled for two solid weeks. Although I did not bleed excessively after my gallbladder operation, the surgery was something I did not want to repeat anytime soon. I am a person who procrastinates and avoids any kind of invasive surgery since the sight of my own blood actually frightens me. I could never be a nurse! Of course, I have the highest admiration for nurses. My three daughters are finicky, too, about any kind of health aftercare, yet they became Florence Nightingale, No. 1, 2, and 3 after my heart surgery September 4, 2003.

I changed doctors in 1998 because two of my daughters, Marlene, and Joyce, were raving about their family physician and how compassionate, brilliant and kind he was, and they thought he could help me with my digestive distress. My records were transferred and my first visit was scheduled, but this young doctor died suddenly from leukemia. I never even met him, thus I was seen by one of his female associates who moved out of town within a year. I drifted from one doctor to another in the group for several years, like a tumble weed in the desert, until I switched to Dr. Altuglu, again because my youngest daughter, Joyce, raved about how knowledgeable she was.

Dr. Altuglu has kept track of my cholesterol and triglycerides, and vital statistics, for several years now, and I attribute her for saving my life. This is how it happened.

Never having smoked cigarettes in my life, exercising with both land and water aerobics since I was in my thirties, hiking for twenty years, and walking and keeping busy, may have prolonged my life. Nevertheless, I was a walking time bomb, which I found out two months ago after a routine visit to Dr. Altuglu. She listened to my heart, and said, “Everything is fine.” I stood up to leave. As I started walking toward the door, I casually mentioned that I noticed I was extra tired lately, and felt like wilted celery, after doing one hour of vigorous water aerobics. I am not sure why I mentioned this on that particular day, because water aerobics has always made me sleepy and extra tired, especially on the occasional days that I had arisen early, around 4:30 AM or so. I was rather surprised when she remarked, “Get up on the table and I will do an EKG.” She noticed some variance in the EKG compared to one taken years ago, and suggested that I have a stress test.

I told Dr. Altuglu that I could not walk on a treadmill because of my inner ear imbalance which I have lived with since I was forty-seven years old. This 16% imbalance and loss of hearing in my left ear was the result of a virus, and my body has swayed like a pendulum ever since. I often hesitate to tell doctors about it because some of them may think I am ridiculous saying that, but I have adjusted to this imbalance and do not notice it very often. Of course, I do feel a little dizzy at times if my stomach is upset. Sometimes, although not often, my world spins around like a top, and I must rest for several hours.

Dr. Altuglu explained that I could have a chemical stress test instead, a test which was performed two months later at Cuyahoga Falls General Hospital. Although it was somewhat uncomfortable, it wasn't anything about which to complain. Two hours later, the heart specialist said, "Everything looks normal!" I was elated at the good news and again resumed my busy daily activities. However, a week later, I received a phone call from Dr. Narraway that there was some damage to my heart. Dr. Narraway happened to be the same doctor who told me that everything looked normal the day of the stress test. His nurse set up an appointment for me. At the visit, Dr. Narraway told me that I was a fifty-fifty patient; that is, I could decide if I wanted to have an angiogram (or catheterization) which might result in an angioplasty.

Being a procrastinator about any type of invasive procedures, I told him that I would think about it. After all, I was planning to fly to Kansas on July 21 - 28 to visit my daughter, Cindy Odom, and her family. Since Cindy teaches fifth grade, it was feasible to travel during July. We planned to see the sights in Missouri and Arkansas.

Three days after I arrived in Kansas, Cindy and her husband, Larry, and I drove to Eureka Springs, Arkansas to see the Passion play. We then drove back to Branson, Missouri to see two wholesome family shows. Larry drove his car and was a great tour guide since he was a native of Kansas and also, at times, worked in Missouri. He showed us his mother's birthplace, some historic landmarks, his grandfather's place, and did it all with a tremendous sense of humor.

I had some stomach distress throughout the trip, but had no chest pains, even when we had been traveling and walking all day. After the Passion play, we did ascend about what seemed like a hundred steps and I felt a little shaky and was somewhat short of breath, but attributed it to my age, spinal stenosis, and the fact that we had been on the go from eight o'clock in the morning until midnight. After we checked into the hotel, I slept all night, and we spent another fun filled day seeing a Broadway show and the Jim Stafford show.

On the way home the next morning, we stopped at Precious Moments and toured the chapel and grounds. There were angels, statues and paintings, everywhere. It was a very enjoyable trip.

After arriving back in Kansas, Cindy and I took a walk or hike each day, went to lunch and shopped. We also visited her son, Shaun, twenty-one years old, and a pre-med student at Kansas University. He showed us the lab where he was doing experimental research on arrythmias with rabbits. We were a little shocked by this method using cute little rabbits, but realized that research must be done to help find new methods of treatment.

We took Shaun out to lunch at an open air restaurant and discussed my heart issues. Shaun remarked, "Grandma, you have to get the angiogram because it will show the correct extent of the damage or blockage in your arteries." Shaun had previously witnessed six angiograms. I decided to listen to him.

Arriving home safely, I called Dr. Narraway to set up the angiogram. In the meantime, our son, Bob, who lives in Texas, E-mailed me and suggested that I could get an MRI heart and lung scan which was not invasive.

A second call to the doctor set up the heart/lung scan at Akron General Hospital. Joyce, our youngest daughter, drove me there. It was an easy test, but it showed a 50% blockage, and two 25% blocked arteries, which we found out later was not correct.

A Bizarre Day as an Outpatient

Shaun and Dr. Narraway again suggested that I have the catheterization, and this time I finally agreed. On August 28 at six AM, my husband went with me to City Hospital where I had the most bizarre experience one can imagine.

As I was entering the preparatory room as an Outpatient, a nurse called me over and asked me to sign some papers. Because I can only see close with my glasses, I never walk with them on and use them only for reading. I took the nurse's word for it that these were my papers, and signed on the dotted line. However, when she announced that a Dr. Larue would be doing my angiogram, I knew something was amiss.

I replied, "That is not right, because Dr. Narraway was supposed to do it."

The nurse said, somewhat sarcastically, "Well, you don't have to do it if you don't want to."

I quickly found my glasses in my purse, and realized that I had signed my name for someone else's procedure. The nurse apologized many times, and said she had never before made that mistake. The woman whose papers I had signed arrived just then, and she was issued new papers.

During the catheterization, which was invasive but did not hurt, I could see the blockages on the screen and it was not a pleasing sight. Dr. Narraway explained that the blockage was too extensive to perform an angioplasty. He remarked, "I have bad news—your right artery is blocked 100% in two spots, and your left arteries are also blocked in two spots, one at 95%, and two at 90%. You will have to have quadruple heart bypass surgery."

Because I could tell from looking at the screen that some of my arteries were completely or almost completely blocked, I was not too shocked at the diagnosis. I asked Dr. Narraway if he would perform the bypass. He answered, "Honey, you wouldn't want me to do it. I will get you the best cardiac surgeon in Akron, Dr. Eric Espinal."

I replied, "Thank you."

The second bizarre incident occurred after I was moved from the room. My daughter, Joyce, joined me as I came out from having the angiogram. A designated person pushed the bed I was on 'lickety split' down the surgical halls. There was a slight incline and she let go of my bed. I wondered why I was traveling so fast, like a roller coaster accelerating. Joyce was behind her and was ready to catch the bed if the person did not. Naturally, we reported this person as soon as we arrived at the outpatient recovery section. The nurses were dismayed that anyone would do such a thing.

Are you ready for what happened next? Joyce left to move her car, and to call Cindy on her cell phone in Overland Park, Kansas, and Marlene at work at FedEx in Fairlawn. Cell phones are not permitted in the surgical areas. As I was being lifted from the bed to another in the recovery room, blood started spurting out of my right groin where the catheter had been inserted. The nurse said, "Oh, no, this never happens."

I thought to myself, *"Never say never."*

Dottie, the very kind nurse who took care of me in the outpatient room, held her hands down tight over the small incision for at least ten minutes. After her arms tired, she asked another nurse to apply pressure for another ten minutes. When the ten pound sand bag was applied over the groin, which is a usual procedure, I felt my bladder needs, and asked for a bed pan. Dottie kindly obliged, pulled the curtain and left. After about five minutes, I pushed on the buzzer to call Dottie, but no one answered my call. I repeatedly pushed the buzzer to no avail, so called out, "Is anybody out there?" Just about that moment, both of my daughters arrived, heard me, and went to get Dottie. Dottie did not hear the buzzer. I thought perhaps it was not working, and I was right. Dottie called the electricians who appeared shortly afterwards to repair or replace the buzzer. I was moved to another room.

Another slight mishap occurred when I ordered some cream of wheat and a cup of hot tea, and was brought cream of wheat and hot coffee which I never drink. That happened twice, breakfast and lunch.

Marlene went back to work, so Joyce and I waited for Doctor Espinal until five PM. I was surprised that he was so young. Joyce and I thought it was quite a coincidence when we found out that he is her gynecologist's husband.

Barb, Dr. Espinal's young nurse, introduced herself and set up the time for my quadruple heart bypass surgery on September 4. Joyce asked Dr. Espinal if I would be able to wait for a week to have the operation, and the doctor said, "Yes." He explained that some small arteries behind my heart had taken over for the main blockage. He also told us that I have a strong heart muscle, and there was no damage to it. That was good news!

After arriving home at about 5:30 PM, I resumed my regular routine, but blood kept seeping through the bandage overnight. I called Dr. Altuglu's office and canceled my September 5 and September 12 appointments for a CBC (complete blood count) and follow up office visit. Dr. Altuglu suggested that I take it easy until the surgery.

However, there was so much to do, such as paying bills, buying groceries, getting my E-check and license plates renewed, preparing meals for my husband, and notifying relatives and THE POET'S NOOK group that I would not be conducting the September 10th meeting. All of my friends and relatives were shocked at hearing the bad news (or good, whichever way you look at it). It was a God-incidence, I believe, that this problem was discovered in time before I had a massive heart attack, and I attributed Dr. Altuglu for saving my life, for she did not ignore my passing remark.

After our Dodge Stratus passed the E-check two days before my surgery, I went to the Bureau of Motor Vehicles to renew my license plates, bought groceries, and prepared some dinners for my husband, Bob, to eat while I was in the hospital. There was not much time to notify everyone, but I wrote or E-mailed some of my relatives to remind them to get an EKG because of our family's genetic history.

September 4, 2003 and Hospital Stay

Bob and I arrived at the outpatient entrance at City Hospital at five AM on September 4, 2003. He stayed with me until I was prepared for the surgery which had been scheduled at seven AM. There was some delay, so the operation was not performed until 9 AM.

I remember entering the operating room thinking, *"What a small table—I hope I don't fall off,"* as they moved me onto it. I looked around and could see my doctor and several of his assistants whom I later met. They all looked so young and I felt that I was in good hands as I said a quick prayer for God to help guide their hands. That's the last thing I remembered until feeling a respiratory tube in my throat four hours later.

At one o'clock, Dr. Espinal spoke to my family and told them I was recovering in the Intensive Care Unit. Our two daughters, Marlene and Joyce, came in to see me, but I do not remember that.

Joyce remarked to Marlene, our sentimental daughter, "Don't you dare cry, for you will make me cry." Marlene, although she is emotional, also has a terrific sense of humor. She had told me several times in the past years, "Mom, you can't ever leave us—we need you too much. But when you do go, I will have to jump in the casket with you!"

Guess who started to cry? Joyce, the usually strong one; so they were both crying when they saw me with all the tubes connected to my body. Marlene panicked, "Mom looks dead," but breathed a sigh of relief as Joyce assured her that I was breathing since she saw the blanket moving up and down.

It took five more hours for the nurse to remove the respiratory tube, although someone kept saying at intervals, "The tube will be removed soon." I felt rather calm and tried to breathe normally.

I was kept in ICU for three days because there were no rooms available on the fourth floor, which was the cardiac floor. While there, I looked forward to having my own room.

My hemoglobin went down to five when it should have been thirteen. I was given two pints of blood through my IV.

One incident that happened in ICU is rather comical. My teeth are very important to me and I have to take special care of them because six years ago I almost lost them to gum disease. While I was sitting up after eating lunch the second day in ICU, I was flossing my teeth. I had been told repeatedly by my periodontist to brush and floss after every meal. A young male nurse or intern, I am not sure which, walked by and exclaimed, "I have never seen anyone flossing their teeth in ICU."

I retorted, more or less in a whisper, "Well, now you have."

I was amazed that I seemed to feel no real pain, just some discomfort in my chest. However, I was plagued with digestive problems which were accelerated perhaps by the shock of the surgery to my whole being. I took all the meds given me and felt that they were upsetting my stomach even more. There were tubes and wires all over me. However, I tried not to notice them. One was even in my neck to draw blood. That tube stayed in until the day I was discharged.

Late on Saturday, I was moved to the cardiac floor, and it was much more comfortable than being in ICU. There was a large window beside the bed which allowed the sunshine to permeate the room, like a warm blanket of cheer.

The nurses were all kind and most of them had a good sense of humor. Unfortunately, I did not sleep well and could not get out of bed by myself partly because of my spinal stenosis, my bandaged leg, and the general weakness one experiences after surgery. To my chagrin, I was told that I could not turn over to sleep on my side. While on my back, it seemed that I kept sliding down in the bed which resulted in very uncomfortable positions.

I was fortunate in that I experienced no pain while in the hospital, except for extreme gastritis, which was probably masking any other discomfort. Of course, there was one incident of pain when an intern pulled a tube from my chest. We called this young intern Dr. Spaghetti, because her last name sounded like 'spaghetti'. She was young, bubbly and kind, and was very popular with everyone on the fourth floor. I thought I remembered her lovely brown eyes looking out from her mask in the operating room, although I was not sure it was her.

Many people, family and friends, visited me each day and brought gifts, flowers, plants, and balloons. Our daughters visited daily; our son, David, who lives in Massillon, visited me once. Our other son, Bob, who lives in Texas, sent four beautiful plants in a very large basket. The plants caught the attention of most visitors. All of the company helped the time pass rather quickly. From midnight until four AM, though, I watched the clock, minute by minute.

My stay was brightened by a visit from our eighteen year old granddaughter, Nikki, who drove home two and a half hours from Bowling Green State University in Ohio to see me that weekend. She brought me a cute BGSU teddy bear and balloons.

One night, after I had fallen asleep at eleven PM, I was awakened at midnight. A nurse instructed me to breathe through an apparatus which looked like a 'peace pipe'. It was given to patients to keep their lungs clear. I never went back to sleep again because I had taken milk of magnesia earlier and my stomach was churning like a washing machine. However, I did not bother the nurses until four AM when the hospital seemed to awaken. Sometimes, after four AM, I fell asleep in the chair or walked the halls with a nurse's help. The third day, while sitting in the chair, I wrote a poem called, NO ONE SLEEPS ON THIS FLOOR, inspired by a remark of one of the nurses after I told her I couldn't sleep.

Here is the poem:

NO ONE SLEEPS ON THIS FLOOR
Floriana Hall

After open heart bypass surgery,
Be it double, triple or quadruple,
The recovery is much faster
Because the nurses harass you.

Nag, nag, nag, they remind you,
Hold your Mended Heart pillow tight,
Don't push up on your arms,
Your habit, with much might.

They wake you up at midnight
When you are sound asleep,
You can't put up a good fight,
So cooperate without a peep.

They poke, listen and make you smile,
They straighten up the bed,
They help you endure indignities
And give you many meds.

These young Florence Nightingales
Work hard all night and day,
Changing bandages, helping you walk,
Listening to nonsense you seem to say.

And no one gets much sleep
When patients must lay on their back,
Thank God for these young caretakers,
They're life savers, that's a fact!

I gave this poem to the nurses on the cardiac floor, and thought they would like it.

Needless to say, hospitals are not my favorite place to be, but I had such good care, I did not complain.

The day before I was discharged, a briefing was given in the lounge room right next to mine. A nurse rescued me from bed just before it started, and I greeted everyone (about twelve people) as I entered. I don't think one person said hello, and most of them frowned like great stone faces.

As I sat down in a comfortable chair, a woman next to me did ask, "How are you?"

I answered, "Fine, thanks, how are you?"

I realized some of these patients were in physical pain and their relatives who were there with them were sharing it. It seemed I was the only person who asked questions of Barb, the nurse giving the presentation. As I left, I said, "I hope all of you recover soon." I did not hear anyone acknowledge that statement.

Our eldest daughter, Cindy, flew to Cleveland from Kansas City on Monday, and all three daughters came to see me on Monday evening. It was so good to see Cindy, too. She took a week off from teaching fifth grade to take care of me. That same evening, one of my poet friends, whose 95 year old father was on the fourth floor, came to see me. She brought me a pink spotted leopard attached to a balloon's ribbon and I treasured it. Her mother, also a poet, was unable to be there that evening.

Homeward bound—September 9, 2003

The next morning, Tuesday, September 9, I was released early by Dr. Espinal. Cindy and my husband came to take me home. Barb took out the last tube in my neck, and changed the bandages on my left leg where the veins were removed. One of the incisions on the side of my left knee was bleeding, but Barb thought that exposing it to air might stop it. On the way home, I sat in the back seat of our car in case of an accident which could cause the air bags to inflate. That would be dangerous after the surgery. I had been told that I would have to be chauffeured for six weeks.

Cindy took excellent care of me. We started to call her, "Florence Nightingale." She was also Betty Crocker, Tillie the hairdresser, and the laundress all rolled into one. She spent a lot of time in the kitchen preparing nutritious meals and freezing them for the next few weeks. She knew her Dad relies on me to cook, and I was told not to do much of anything for the first two weeks, at least.

The next day, my leg incision started to bleed again, and quite heavily. Dr. Espinal had said that it was "old blood." We took turns applying pressure on the wound with gauze, and it took an hour to slow it down to a minimum. Bob, at one point, almost fell asleep while holding the gauze. We found out later that his blood pressure was too low, 92 over 52, and that explained why he seemed to be so sleepy. His doctor then told him not to take his blood pressure medication, and a week later, his blood pressure was normal.

The next week was filled with company; wonderful friends, neighbors and family visiting. It helped pass the time because time seemed to go so slowly for me, as it does for probably everyone who is recuperating from heart surgery. A neighbor brought homemade noodle soup, a friend brought an apple pie and pumpkin bread, another friend, blueberry muffins, so we had plenty of food.

Taking showers seemed like such a chore and tired everyone. You see, I was still a little nauseous and dizzy, so going down stairs to take a shower made me extra wobbly. The shower in the upstairs bathroom was not working properly, and I was told not to take a tub bath for six weeks or more, until my leg wounds healed. Bob and Cindy helped me down the stairs so that I would not fall. How I missed the warm tub baths and the whirlpool! As I mentioned before, water, as well as water aerobics and tub baths, have always made me tired and sleepy, but showers did not really result in the same cozy feeling.

Cindy, (and later Marlene and Joyce), handed me, one at a time, three washcloths and three towels as needed, while I held on to the shower bar. Each incision had to be washed and dried separately, while the third set of towels was used to dry the rest of my body. I actually took my first shower at Joyce's home because it is a ranch style with everything on one floor. Unfortunately, my leg bled on her carpet, but I was relieved that she was able to get the stain out immediately. After that, all my showers were taken at my own home.

Bob, Cindy and I went to see Dr. Espinal on Friday. As I worked my way out of the car, my leg started to bleed profusely and my Capri pants were drenched with blood. Soon we arrived at the automatic door, which was not working that day. Since we had never been to Dr. Espinal's office before, we asked directions. The directions were incorrect, naturally, and we ended up in the North section of the building. Meanwhile, blood kept dripping on the carpet. I saw a red wheelchair sitting in a corner and promptly sat down in it. Bob pushed the wheelchair and Cindy led us back to the South building. Bob was uptight and I was almost panicky as he pushed me into the elevator hitting my left arm on the side. It was a wild ride!

Dr. Espinal saw me in a few minutes and again reiterated that it was "old blood." His nurse put three stitches in the wound, and we left for home. They gave me some scrubs to wear, for my Capri's and underpants were covered with blood. Since the automatic doors were not working, the wheelchair got stuck on the track, so I quickly stood up because Cindy could not hold the heavy door any longer. It was really good to be back home after that misadventure.

The first night at home, Cindy helped me out of bed when I called her. The second night, something awesome happened. In the hospital, I could not turn over in the narrow bed, but in my own double bed, there was room and I inadvertently must have turned over on my side or stomach in my sleep. I could feel ethereal arms turning me over on my back, and as I was gently plopped on the pillow right side up on my back, I woke up startled. Neither Cindy nor Bob turned me over, so it had to be my guardian angel. I have felt an angel's presence other times in my life. What a marvelous experience it is! This saved me from having possible further surgery. A heart patient is only permitted to sleep on his or her back.

Cindy provided excellent care and neither the girls nor Bob and I wanted her to leave, but she was due back in Kansas to teach her fifth grade students the next Monday. Joyce drove her to the Cleveland airport on Sunday, September 14.

Marlene, 'Florence II', stayed with me for two days and was also an excellent companion. However, the nights were rather unusual after she went home. Bob bought a bell for me to ring to awaken him to help me at night when needed. Unfortunately, the first two nights, he was not awakened by the bell or by my constantly shouting his name. After twenty minutes of waiting to go to the bathroom, I knew I had to get out of bed by myself. However, I was not supposed to push on my elbow to get up. I piled pillows and a quilt behind my back for support, held the Mended Hearts pillow tightly, and prayed that pushing on my elbow would not hurt my progress. This pillow was given to me the first day after surgery, a usual procedure. However, no one ever came in to explain about the Mended Hearts Group which donates them. I learned about them later.

It was now Joyce's turn to help me for three days, and she took excellent care of me, also, and helped with the housework. On Wednesday, September 17, we decided to expose the wound to air and it finally stopped bleeding. When Ann, the visiting nurse came on Thursday, she noticed that my leg was inflamed and hard—it was infected. She called Dr. Espinal and he told me to come in on Friday at the time my regular appointment was scheduled.

Dr. Espinal lanced the two infected incisions on my leg and Barb showed Joyce how to insert the gauze wick and bandage it. I did not feel a thing when Dr. Espinal lanced the incisions, causing blood to spurt out. I could not really see it, since I was lying down on the table. They grimaced as I chatted away, Joyce told me later. Dr. Espinal remarked, "You are an amazing woman, and must have coped with a lot in your life." Later on, I told him about the two books I had written, SMALL CHANGE, and DADDY WAS A BAD BOY, depicting the adversity I lived through as a child.

The doctor then prescribed Levaquin, an antibiotic which I took for weeks. He told me to walk as much as possible.

Joyce dressed my wounds the next day—it was a tedious thing to do. Because I was still so pale and weak, the visiting nurses came to change the bandages twice a day for a week or more.

I had wondered why I looked so ghostly and ghastly in the bathroom mirror since arriving home from the hospital and why I was occasionally seeing double when reading or watching television. After mentioning this to Ann, the visiting nurse, she told me that anesthesia can do that to your vision for about two months and she suggested that I should not have my eyes examined until November if I wanted a correct diagnosis. She also told me that the reason my pinkies were going to sleep was because of the anesthesia.

On Sunday, September 21, Ann thought that my leg looked worse, so she called Dr.Espinal, who suggested that I be taken to the Emergency Room at City Hospital. Marlene took me there, where an intern checked me immediately, but did nothing since I was to see Dr. Espinal the next day.

The same day that I visited ER, our granddaughter, Nikki, was stung by a bee inside her dorm at Bowling Green State University. She started to swell and noticed two streaks traveling up her arm. At midnight, another former Tallmadge High School student drove her to the ER at the hospital in Bowling Green. Nikki was told that she was allergic to bee venom and given steroids, an antibiotic, Benydryl and Pepcid. No one told her to eat a snack with all that medication, thus she was awake all night with an upset stomach and dizziness. I felt badly about her being allergic to bees, like I am, for now she would have to avoid them, just like I do. I have been running away from bees for about fifteen years. At times, when walking in the park, several bees have hovered above my head at once, and I am continually avoiding them during the bee season.

Ann, the visiting nurse, and I were talking the next morning, September

22, and she told me that her five year old twins were stung at camp over the weekend.

During Joyce's lunch hour that afternoon, she drove me to Dr. Espinal's office. When Dr. Espinal walked in and overheard us discussing bees, he told us he was stung while coaching his son's soccer team. Bees were obviously numerous this particular time of year.

Joyce took me to Dr. Espinal's office once again on September 26, at which time he thought that my leg looked somewhat better. He encouraged me to walk at the mall.

Heart patients are required to walk ten minutes, four times a day, the first six weeks. I did walk at the mall with a neighbor friend several times, and with Joyce and Bob, too. But mostly, I walked around the house in circles for ten minutes at a time from one room to another. I also did all of the arm and leg exercises required, did my breathing exercises, and ate nutritiously.

Writing consumed some of my time, but I was eager to get to the six weeks date, October 16, when I could drive once again. Bob seemed to have a heavy foot and hit all of the bumps everywhere we went.

Thankfully, at this point, I was feeling well enough to resume some enjoyable activities. Bob and I went to see a movie, called SECONDHAND LIONS, the third week of my recuperation. Joyce brought food over for us many times, and took me to church the fifth week. I had watched the Mass on television the first four Sundays, but was relieved to get back to the actual services. Finally, after the sixth week, I drove to Mass by myself. During the recuperation period, I wrote two more poems. Here is the second poem:

BLESSINGS LIKE A FOUNTAIN
Floriana Hall

Give me my teddy bears, my pink leopard and my angel
And I will get well soon
Give me my Mended Heart pillow and I'll hug it, too.
Give me courage and strength to cope with each day
Whatever befalls, triumphs or setbacks along the way.
Shower me with blessings like a fountain
Help me to trek slowly over mountains,
Give me faith, hope and charity
Let me see things clearly and be tolerant
Give me patience to listen and learn

Close my ears to babbling obscenities
Open my heart to love and kindness
Close my mouth to any negatives,
Open my mind to absorb the goodness
Like a sponge drawing up moisture
Or a wick sucking out infection.
Fill me with grace and let me pray
To thank the good Lord every day.
Let me feel the Angel lift me
Turn me over when I can't.
Give me family, friends and foresight,
Let me be there for them when needed,
Hold their hand and whisper love words.
Let me inhale the fragrance
Of each beautiful flower
Sprinkled with morning dew
Let me taste of honey and lemons
Let this stream spurt life anew.
And the jet will wash away sorrow
Pain, loneliness and ailments
Touching others with tenderness
A spring of compliant contentment.

Floriana Hall—September 21, 2003

Dr. Espinal set up an appointment for me on October 10. In the meantime, the visiting nurses came once a day instead of twice, and I learned to dress my wounds myself. Gradually, as one of the wounds closed up, the nurses visited twice a week. Finally, on October 17, the second wound began to close and I could use a Band Aid instead of the bulky bandages that caused my legs to look raw and wrinkled because of the tape.

My last visit to Dr. Espinal was on October 24, 2003, when he pronounced that it would be the last time I would have to see him. He surprised me by reciting a poem he had written when he was in high school. That is when I told him more about my books and poetry. I would miss him and his assistants. One of his assistants told me that he was happy to have patients like me who smiled and were happy instead of grumpy old people. That was gratifying to hear. I would rather miss Dr. Espinal, his assistants, and the visiting nurses, but I was glad to be dismissed.

Here is the third poem I wrote:

ALIVE AGAIN
Floriana Hall

It's good to be alive
Not merely just survive
To inhale fresh autumn air
See leaves falling with a flair.

Six weeks of sitting there—
A comfortable chair,
But inactivity is not me
Creativity's fashion carefree.

Using hands, not just my mind,
Using feet to walk streamlined
Turning, bending, pushing, pulling
Doing housework, even grueling.

To be myself again,
To satisfy a yen,
Life's winter season
Enjoyed with reason.

I'll taste of milk and honey
I'll laugh at something funny,
I'll catch the first snow
Leave footprints below.

I'll behold spring flowers
Climb ivory towers
Hug all my kin
Have joy within.

Summer sun will be jolly
Nostalgia melancholy,
Then when autumn comes again
I'll say, "I made it, Amen."

Most of all, I will pray
Thank God every day
For the gift of being here
With friends and family dear.

Floriana Hall—October 19, 2003

You might think that this is the end of the story, but not so. Since I had suggested that all of my relatives consider having an EKG, my brother, Frank, who is 72 years old, did just that. He did not have symptoms at the time, but a few weeks later, felt some kind of gurgling in his chest after he chopped wood while building a deck. An angiogram was done on Wednesday, October 22, and it was found out that Frank had 100% blockage in his main artery, and 70% in several others, plus a leaky heart valve and an enlarged heart. He was kept in the hospital and on October 24 a quadruple heart bypass was performed. The leaky heart valve was also repaired. Veins were taken out of both of his legs. I waited most of the day with his family in the Central Lounge at City Hospital. At four PM, his doctor announced that the surgery was over and he would be fine.

Frank felt weak like I did at first, but looked better on October 29, 2003. Bob and I visited him just before the ambulance was to take him to an aftercare facility.

It is ironic that this same surgery would be performed on brother and sister within seven weeks. But thank God we found out in time. I hope to help other people realize that it is important to get an EKG or stress test even without any symptoms of heart disease.

REHAB—December 2003

When I was finally released for rehabilitation, I found out that the sessions were held at various times on Monday, Tuesday, and Thursday. At first I joined a 10:30 AM class, but three weeks later was transferred to a 2:00 PM class because it was better suited to my busy schedule.

I informed the nurses that I could not walk on the treadmill because of my inner ear imbalance, so I kept busy on the other machines. After two weeks using the arm machine, I developed bursitis is my right shoulder, which I had had once years before. That was the first real pain I experienced since the operation. Needless to say, I did not use the arm machines any more.

One day while exercising on the bicycle, someone tapped me on the shoulder, and I was surprised to see my brother, Frank, there for orientation. He was feeling much better since he had been taken off a blood thinner, which had to be measured constantly. He had a tissue valve replacement and had some fibrillation problems, besides the quadruple bypass, and that is why he was put on Coumadin.

I had many misadventures at rehab, also, so wrote a poem about the funny incidents. Here it is:

MISADVENTURES OF REHAB
Floriana Hall

**When the cold chill air of winter
Creeps into these brittle old bones,
I want to curl up in a blanket and simmer
Like cocoa to drink with scones.**

**Oh, but wait, I can't eat scones
For they are full of fat
Chocolate does not agree with my system,
Fiddledeedee and drat!**

**Instead of keeping warm and toasty
I must venture out in this frigid season
To exercise on stationery bikes
To keep on living is the reason.**

**Arm machines are difficult to turn
They bring on some bursitis,
Stair climbing apparatus strains
And brings on spinal arthritis.**

The drive there consists of detours
Construction is everywhere,
I'm not that fond of driving
But nobody seems to care.

I can't even reach the ticket
When I arrive at the gate,
I have to get out of the car,
FREE parking could make me late.

One day when I was leaving
The gate would not open at all,
The machine had eaten my ticket,
I was trapped, I wanted to bawl.

What to do but keep on going
And doing what I must—
There's no choice in this matter
Requiring exercise, one thing I trust.

That it will help my heart,
My whole body to renew,
I'll get back to aerobics in water
To enjoy other than my brew.

Meanwhile, the people are friendly,
I'm starting to like this place,
It's good to learn something new
A different concept to embrace.

Floriana Hall—December 16, 2003

A week later, I noticed that someone had knocked down the gate entrance. Perhaps someone had been trapped as I was the first week I went there. It was rather comical, although, in reality, destructive.

When I was half way finished with rehab, the weather turned really nasty, with one snowstorm after another, followed by an ice storm the likes of which

I had never before seen. A week before the ice storm, my husband had fallen on the sidewalk while shoveling snow. Although he had turned eighty two years old on January 15, 2004, he was still very active. However, he bruised his shoulder and ribs on his left side and was in a great deal of pain for several weeks after the fall. We were iced in for a few days, and I missed one day of rehab.

It was time to see Dr. Altuglu again. My cholesterol and triglycerides were elevated somewhat since the last visit, so she prescribed a new cholesterol lowering medication that had proven not to have many side effects. When I tried Crestor the next day, it seemed to agree with me.

After I arrived home from the doctor's visit, Bob came upstairs and staggered twice, and fell on the kitchen floor. He lay there for about ten minutes, and finally, I was able to help him up from a sitting position. His 240 pounds was more weight than I can handle, so the whole day was filled with stress. After questioning him, I found out that he had taken a whole day's supply of medication at once while I was gone, and had not eaten anything. He rested most of that day, and I prayed for him that night. Thankfully, the next day he felt better, so I pleaded with him never to take all his pills all at once without eating. I decided to monitor the pill situation after that incident.

During the first week of February, the weather in Akron was still very cold, with sleet and snow build up on the side streets and driveways. Bob was still recuperating from his falls outdoors and indoors, so was unable to chip the ice from our driveway. As a result, on February 4, as I was returning from a club meeting, and driving slowly up our driveway, the front passenger wheel on my 2001 Dodge Stratus slid into our window well. I was totally surprised by the sudden plunge, and hurried into the house to call a tow truck. Because of the neighbor's air conditioner and fence in the way, the tow truck could not pull my car out of the window well except from behind. Thus the car was damaged to the extent of $607, which was covered partly by our insurance.

I drove a loaner car for three days until my car was repaired. While going to rehab during that time, I could not help but chuckle once again because the gate entrance was down for the third time. One could tell that someone had deliberately run the gate down because that person had been trapped in the entrance.

As Valentine's Day approached, I was told that my last day of rehab would be Monday, February 16. Medicare paid only for 36 sessions, and because of Thanksgiving, Christmas, and New Year's Day off, I had fulfilled the commitment somewhat earlier. I had missed three other days, two while our family members were here from out of town for the holidays, and one during the ice storm.

Although I was accustomed to going to rehab, and enjoyed the people there and even the machines, I felt relieved, like a weight lifted off my shoulders. From February 16 on, I was able to come and go as I chose, and return to water aerobics when ready. Of course, I will always exercise, for I know it is the best way to keep my heart and body healthy.

One thing that I noticed after my return to water aerobics was the fact that the water exercise still made me sleepy and tired, and I needed a nap sometime during the day or evening, just like before the surgery.

So many people have told me that they think I look great for having had the bypass, and I tell them that it is prayer and the grace of God that helped me. Actually, sometimes I feel like I never had quadruple heart bypass surgery, or that I am a person with heart disease. I mentioned this to Dr. Narraway on my June 2004 six month visit, and he replied, "That is good, and it is also bad in some respects." I questioned him as to what he meant by that, and he replied, "It is good that you are feeling so well, but it could be bad if you forget to follow the right eating patterns." I assured him that I would never do that, except for chocolate.

He then told me that I did not have to return for another appointment for a year, and that I was doing super. What a blessing it was to hear that, although, as I stated above, I feel like I never had surgery or heart disease.

JOANN SCHINDLER'S HISTORY OF HEART DISEASE

When JoAnn was seven years old and in the second grade of school, she started coughing constantly, so her mother took her to the coal mining company doctor where her father worked. He treated her for bronchitis, but she continued to cough.

A short time later, JoAnn and her mother visited her mother's sister in Pittsburgh, who suspected that something else was wrong. JoAnn's aunt called her pediatrician and he immediately sent JoAnn to Allegheny General Hospital in Pittsburgh. An X-ray of her heart was taken and the cardiologist said that her heart was very enlarged and inflamed. The diagnosis was rheumatic fever. JoAnn was given oral penicillin in liquid form daily while she stayed in a hospital closer to her home for six weeks. She felt very ill during this time. But, since she was an obedient and easy going child, she did not seem to mind the long stay. She was happy to play with her dolls, and she enjoyed drinking chocolate milk every day at the hospital.

After JoAnn was released from the hospital, she spent a year in bed to rest her heart muscle and to strengthen it. The year went by more quickly than she thought it would, and soon she was back in school. However, JoAnn's heart remained large and she also had atrium fibrillation.

Going back to school seemed traumatic for little JoAnn, who was placed in the third grade. She thought it was difficult to keep up because she had missed so much. Since she was behind in reading, her parents enrolled her in three different schools trying to help her. When JoAnn was ten years old, one of her teachers noticed that she was lip reading, so began to tutor her. With the help of this devoted teacher, JoAnn eventually became fluent in reading.

JoAnn graduated from high school and obtained a secretarial job at B & W in Barberton. Shortly afterwards, she met her future husband who was a native Akronite. At first, JoAnn was a little hesitant about getting married, and was not sure why. Perhaps she had a premonition that her heart would cause some problems during her lifetime. However, they did marry and had two children. They had a good marriage.

One day, while she was on her way to work, she became extremely tired. She started coughing up blood in the parking lot, and went into the ladies' rest room where this process continued. Immediately after contacting a cardiologist, he admitted her to the hospital for a catheterization test. The test revealed that her mitral valve was ninety percent closed, and she had heart arrhythmia.

JoAnn belonged to Jehovah's Witness, a faith which did not approve of the heart lung machine because, at that time, it was primed with blood. Members of Jehovah's Witness believe that taking blood into one's body through the mouth or veins violates God's laws, and they cite Genesis 9:3, 4; Leviticus 17:14; Acts 15:28, 29 from Bible scripture as their source.

In 1963, Joanne's doctor performed surgery using another method to get into the heart, rather than the heart lung machine. He opened up the defective valve using his finger. After that, JoAnn was advised to take Lanoxin to help with her atrium fibrillation.

When JoAnn was forty-four years old, she noticed that she was extremely tired and could hardly keep up with her household duties and the stress of two teenagers. She had previously requested that a catheterization test be done. Because she was pre menopausal, the doctors decided to delay it because they knew it might cause a bleeding problem during her menstrual period. About that time, JoAnn's mother informed her that when she was a young child, the doctor did not expect her to live beyond five years. JoAnn wished that her mother had told her that years ago.

However, in 1986, it was time for the mitral valve to be replaced. The heart lung machine was now primed with saline solution, making it possible for her to have open heart surgery without a blood transfusion After the replacement, she was put on Coumadin. Because of continued excessive bleeding during her menstrual period, JoAnn had a total hysterectomy in 1989.

In the year 2000, she began having new problems and gained about 35 pounds from fluid buildup and was found to be in heart failure. After the cardiologist's visit, he decided to take her off Lanoxin because he thought it was toxic to her brain, resulting in depression. JoAnn started to feel better, became more active and lost the extra weight.

However, in 2003, she started filling up with fluid again because of tricuspid valve failure. Her stomach was extended and she had peripheral edema because of the water weight. She was told to take 80 mg of Lasix a day. She was still very tired, resulting in depression once more.

After she consulted with her cardiologist again, JoAnn herself suggested that it was time for a heart catheterization to find out exactly what was going on with her heart. During the procedure, it was found that the tricuspid valve needed repair. The surgery was scheduled for August 4, 2003, but was postponed because JoAnn's hemoglobin was only ten. She took Epogen shots for three months to build up her red blood cells, in order to prepare her for bloodless surgery, which was performed August 29, 2003. It was discovered, because of the position of the mitral and tricuspid valve, that she would need a pacemaker.

Her cardiologist performed the surgery and everything went perfectly fine. Before the surgery, he had told JoAnn that she was a very sick person when he first met her, and that, if she had not had the surgery, she most likely would have died within a couple of years.

She was in the hospital seventeen days because it took three days to drain the fluid from her body in order for the surgery to be successful. The doctors waited four days to install the pacemaker. JoAnn's heart was beating 55 beats a minute, so this procedure was absolutely necessary.

JoAnn recuperated and finished the rehabilitation exercise program. She felt much better afterwards. While she was recuperating, her daughter had a baby on February 2, 2004, who is the delight of JoAnn's life.

Throughout the years, prayer was a priority in JoAnn's daily routine. She felt that prayer would strengthen her and help her to maintain a positive attitude. Her congregation and friends also prayed for her. She continues to find solace in daily prayer.

(JoAnn passed away on June 14, 2005, after filling up with water following bladder surgery).

PATRICIA ALBANESE'S HEART

Patricia Albanese (Pat) was born on February 8, 1935, into a normal middle class family. Her father, William Bean, worked in a factory, and her mother was a stay at home mom.

When Pat was thirteen, the family doctor, while checking her heart, heard a heart murmur and concluded that she might have had rheumatic fever when she was younger. However, her mother did not think so. Although there were no tests done at that time, she was restricted from playing sports and gym. She was also told to rest every day after school, and thus started reading avidly to pass the time. She read every book she could. In the eighth grade, she read almost all of the books in the school library, her favorite being "The Black Stallion."

Pat's father had a heart murmur when he was forty years old, and went to Dr. Ormand, a heart specialist. When Pat was eighteen, she decided to make an appointment with Dr. Ormand, at which time he did an EKG. Because of her heart murmur, Dr. Ormand suggested that she should not plan to have too many children when she got married.

Patricia and Charles A. Albanese were married on November 15, 1958, and subsequently, they had four sons. During her pregnancies, Dr. Flynn, an internal medicine specialist, watched Pat very carefully. He suggested that she have a catheterization of her heart, but she declined because she was leery about the test. Someone had told Charles that it was a horrible test.

After each delivery, Pat's heart murmur quieted down. She was given penicillin every day after her second son was born to protect her heart from staph and other infections. She also took penicillin when she had dental work done.

After taking penicillin for twenty years, it was discovered that bacteria were becoming resistant to penicillin and other antibiotics. Pat was told to stop taking penicillin when she was about 46 years old.

The family led a fairly normal life, although Pat was careful not to overdo or overexert herself, but probably did sometimes, like most people do.

Charles was very supportive and helped her, as did her parents and her in-laws.

It was discovered that two of their four sons had heart murmurs. One son's was detected at birth and the other son's at age 13.

Life went rather smoothly until Pat was fifty-seven years old. At that time, her brother in California was in a coma from a very serious illness. Pat, Charles, and Pat's mother traveled to California to help take care of him while his wife ran his business. They stayed with them for seven weeks.

The next year, Pat's mother broke her shoulder and moved in with Pat and Charles. After her mother recuperated, all three of them again decided to visit her brother in California. Pat developed a cough, and thought she had bronchitis. She went to the Same Day Center where they x-rayed her lungs. The doctor thought she had developed asthma and gave her an inhaler. While they visited in California, they walked every day. Pat had trouble breathing each time they walked. One very hot afternoon, they climbed up one of the mountains at a park. As they were coming down, Pat noticed that her hands had swollen, puffed up like a marshmallow. She could not understand why.

After arriving back home, Pat could scarcely breathe and was taken to Akron General Hospital Emergency, where she was told she had pneumonia. They gave her some breathing treatments that seemed to help a lot. She went home, but the next day, her breathing was worse. She called the doctor to get permission to go back for more breathing treatments. However, the doctor said she did not have pneumonia, and gave her a prescription for Lasix, which Charles picked up for her. Pat was having difficulty breathing and had to lean over to get her breath. She was apprehensive about Charles leaving in case she felt worse and could not call 911. Just at that moment, their son stopped in and stayed with her for half an hour on his lunch break so Charles could leave to get the prescription.

After taking the pills, Pat lost about five pounds of water by nightfall, and her breathing was back to normal.

Pat's doctor then set up an appointment for her with a heart specialist, who scheduled a catheterization for her in August. In the meantime, Pat and Charles went to Bardstown, Kentucky, for a Bean family reunion. At the reunion, Pat told her darling cousin that she was going to have a heart catheterization and he said, "Patricia, have a monkey heart put in so Chuck can have a lot of fun." That's the kind of sympathy she got!

At a visit after the catheterization, the specialist told her that she had cardiomyopathy and was a good candidate for a heart transplant. When he said that, all Pat could think of was monkey hearts which made her laugh. Pat surmised that he probably thought she was nuts to have such a reaction, but realized people respond differently to diagnoses. The specialist prescribed a medication which subsequently made her cough, so he told her to quit taking it.

Pat was given a different type of medication which she took for about five years. She and her husband dieted, walked, watched their cholesterol, and tried to live a healthy life.

In the spring of 1997, Pat received a gift of a massage and nails at a spa. It was a cold and blustery day when Pat decided to visit the spa. After she entered the building, she noticed that she had heart pains, and thought the weather may have aggravated them. A nurse gave her some nitroglycerin pills which took away the pain. She enjoyed the massage and getting her nails done, but after she drove home, she called her doctor. He advised her to call an ambulance and go to the emergency room at Akron General Medical Center where tests were performed.

Since her former heart specialist retired, Pat had been seeing Dr. Tobias, a family doctor, with whom she talked over extraordinary health measures in case of death. She told him that she and Charles had recently signed the documents for Power of Attorney and a Living Will. Dr. Tobias told her not to worry because he would treat her congestive heart failure very aggressively.

Pat was told to be on a salt less diet, but she found that very hard to do when they ate at a restaurant or someone else's home. One time, when they were in Las Vegas and she ate some bacon, she had difficulty breathing and spent the last day there in a hotel. Although she did not get to see all the sights in that city, she still had a good time. However, on the plane flying home, her breathing was labored again.

When she arrived home, Pat's brother was visiting from California. He took her downtown to see her internal medicine doctor. Meanwhile, he crossed the street to St. Mary's to visit a friend. Her doctor listened to her heart and suggested that they call an ambulance to take her to the hospital. Since they were only a few blocks from the hospital, Pat decided to go there in the car.

Suddenly, the power and lights went off in the building. Pat was put in a wheel chair and wheeled through the lobby. She called St. Mary's. Her brother was not there, for he had come back from his visit and was sitting in the lobby. He actually saw the wheelchair go by and never dreamed it was Pat because he could not see clearly in the dark. However, they finally found each other and drove to the ER. Pat asked the doctor what he heard when he listened to her heart, and he replied that he heard a third sound.

After having another catheterization, Dr. Tobias surmised that Pat might have had a heart attack at some earlier time, but that the current chest pains were caused by a hiatal hernia and not from her heart. He called Dr. Maxwell, a gastroenterologist, who did a test by putting a tube down Pat's throat, which sent her into heart failure. That frightened the doctor and Pat was sent back to the hospital again. Dr. Tobias concluded the pains were not caused by her heart but by acid reflux. After he asked Pat if she wanted a second opinion, she went to the Cleveland Clinic.

Approximately fifteen trips to Akron General Medical Center and the Cleveland Clinic were made in a year and a half to determine that Pat had congestive heart failure. Some appointments were just tests and treatments and some were very hairy. In one incident, Pat called 911 before she awakened her husband because she was having difficulty breathing and had coughed up water. On the trip to the hospital, Pat told the ambulance attendant that she did not think she was going to make it to the hospital and needed some Lasix. However, that seemed to be a big mistake, since the driver stopped and pulled over. He called to get permission to put an IV in Pat's arm. Later on, Pat realized they could have been there much sooner if she had not panicked, but she pulled through, just as she had many times before.

On one ambulance trip, an attendant was trying to position an IV in Pat's arm, and she told him she saw a good vein. He asked "Where?" Pat pointed to a big vein she saw going down his arm. She did not get away with that one!

Pat kept getting worse all the time, and could not walk to the mailbox, approximately 150 feet up the driveway, without getting chest pains.

On one occasion in ER, a male nurse started laughing while he was doing Pat's EKG. Pat asked him what was so funny, and he replied, "The new resident in ER will probably hit the ceiling when he sees your EKG because it showed you are having a full blown heart attack." Pat also laughed while talking with him. When he took the EKG to the new resident, sure enough, the poor guy came running over and called in specialists who took excellent care of Pat.

At one point, Pat went to Akron General Medical Center Cardio Pulmonary for exercise classes, and she enjoyed that very much.

On another occasion, Pat had a very bad night in ICU but a wonderful nurse, Shelley, stayed with her every minute. Two doctors came in to take care of her. She couldn't breathe normally and fought them off as they gave her a shot and put the ventilator down her nose. Before she passed out, she remembered hearing them say that it was coming out of her mouth. The next morning, Pat was on the ventilator when she awakened to see all of her family staring at her. They told her later that she looked scared, but she thought that she was just trying to talk and could not wake up.

Another time when Pat was in the hospital, her primary doctor came to see her accompanied by six or eight doctors. One of them told her that they were going to give her some medicine which would make her feel very strange, but that that feeling would only last a minute. However, Pat really felt terrible! She was told later on that the medicine made her heart stop for thirty seconds. She would have probably refused this particular test if she had known ahead of time how she would have been affected.

On her first visit to the Cleveland Clinic, Pat told her doctors her medical history, including her chest pains, and they said the pains were caused by her heart. She had all kinds of tests and a cat scan, after which the doctors then changed their diagnosis to acid reflux. They sent Pat to their gastroenterologist, who did some tests, but she never heard his opinion. She still had chest pains and was taking nitro pills. This episode made her think that medical diagnosis is not an exact science. She did learn that no matter how sick people are, the patients need to be alert enough to ask questions and speak up for themselves. Still, everyone treated Pat kindly at all times.

While at the Cleveland Clinic, a biopsy was done of Pat's heart. As a small catheter was put into a large vein of her neck, the pressures of all the chambers were checked, and pieces of her heart were taken out. All the while the nurses laughed and joked, Pat was freezing and felt like a nervous wreck. They did tell her that the first heart transplant patient from sixteen years before was still alive and drinking, smoking and stealing cars. That remark made her feel somewhat better for a few minutes.

On May 24, 1998, Pat had a very strange and unusual spiritual experience that cannot be explained. It was Pat's grandson's birthday. That day, St. Matthews's was celebrating the priest's 45th anniversary mass and having a dinner afterwards.

As they were standing at the service shaking hands with everyone around them, Pat suddenly felt an arm around her shoulder and a soft whisper in her ear saying, "Don't worry, don't be afraid." She was standing and talking, so knew she was not dreaming, sleeping or drowsing. In her mind's eye, she thought she saw the back of a tall, thin, bald man, in a long robe. Afterwards, she went to the dinner and to their grandson's birthday party.

The next morning, Pat was in the hospital again. She thought perhaps she had ingested too much salt the day before. She remembered the previous night's experience, which she did not really understand, but took great comfort in those whispered words, "Don't worry, don't be afraid."

In 1998, one of the Cleveland Clinic doctors told Pat that they would check into putting her on the transplant list if she would consider this. Pat told him that she had already been considering the procedure for a long time and knew her answer would be yes. She did ask them what to expect, though. The doctor told her that the average time a transplanted heart lasted was approximately five and three quarters years. That made Pat wonder if it would be worth all the pain and expense of the medications that she would have to take. However, she knew she had a good insurance policy, and that comforted her.

That same afternoon, her grandchildren, Kyle and Carly, came to see Pat. Kyle looked Pat straight in the face with his big brown eyes. While he was talking, Pat started thinking about her grandson, Peter, who wasn't yet one year old. She realized that if she did not have the transplant, she might not get to see him when he turned five years old. That fact immediately changed her mind, and it all seemed worthwhile.

One other time when Pat was in the Emergency Room at Akron General Medical Center, they kept her there for eight hours while trying to transport her to the Cleveland Clinic. At first, they couldn't find an ambulance equipped to take her there. After finally finding one, Pat's husband followed the ambulance to Cleveland. Pat was all wired up and had a special nurse traveling with her.

After arriving at the Cleveland Clinic, Pat was so sick that they would not let her get out of bed for any reason. When weighing her every day, she was rolled onto her side to put a sling net under her, then rolled the other way to scoot the net under her, after which she was lifted into the air to be weighed. They left her hanging there while the nurses changed the bedding. That was probably the most uncomfortable experience Pat could remember. It seemed to her it would have been much easier to get up and stand on the scale. Nevertheless, everyone was pleasant, and Pat had no complaints about the care. She really did not think she would live to go home, but was pleasantly fooled again.

The trips to the Emergency Room were very stressful for Charles, her husband. He was also taking care of the lawn, the housework and the dishes, along with helping Pat's mother. However, Pat was able to cook dinner. To ease everyone's burden, they decided to get some help and hired a lovely girl, Debbie, to come in and clean once a week.

In June 1999, Pat was back in the Cleveland Clinic again. The doctors decided to put in a pacemaker-defibrillator. Pat felt as though she was not going to go home alive and she and Charles discussed her feelings. Fortunately, the doctors pulled her through again. Charles was really nervous about taking Pat home.

The same day Pat left the Cleveland Clinic, Charles' brother, Mike, who had cirrhosis of the liver, went into the hospital to see about a liver transplant. He died there two weeks later at seventy years old, which broke their hearts and added more stress, especially for Charles.

Another traumatic thing happened after they were invited to a family wedding. Pat also was invited to the shower, so Pat and Charles went shopping to buy a gift. Since Pat was not feeling well, she asked the clerk if she could sit down, but there were no chairs. Pat decided to sit on a window sill when, all of a sudden, whoosh, she was shocked and the impact threw her about six feet. Another shock made her realize that it was the defibrillator. She lay down on the floor and asked the clerk to call 911. While people were standing all around her out of curiosity and compassion, Pat experienced two more shocks but tried to calm herself. Someone went to find her mother and another person put a box under her feet. After the ambulance arrived, Charles, along with Pat's mother, followed the ambulance to the hospital.

The transplant was seriously considered. Pat was interviewed by a social worker and a group of doctors who voted for the transplant. After traveling to Cleveland many times, Pat was told in August that she was accepted for the heart transplant. However, sometimes it took a long time to find the right heart because of matching the blood type and size. She was told that they had done ninety-eight transplants in 1998, the year before, and all survived except one person because of other complications. Pat's husband told her that he would agree to anything she decided. Pat chose the transplant because she thought the odds were pretty good. She thought that, after the procedure, she and Charles could travel and enjoy his retirement. She was told she was in good shape for a sixty four year old woman except for her heart. Pat was scheduled to take classes in Cleveland so as to understand what to expect.

Before Pat started taking any classes, they received a phone call at one o'clock in the morning on September 1. They had just arrived home from a visit.

Pat picked up the phone and a nurse said, "Guess what, we have good news for you, we have a heart." This was a complete shock to Pat, and she could hear her husband breathing very hard on the other phone. Pat responded, "I am not ready for this; it was supposed to take a long time." The nurse explained to her that the people in her blood group all needed large hearts except her and this was a small one. She gave Pat half an hour to decide while the doctor was at Metro hospital examining the heart. If it was the right one for Pat, she had only one hour to get to the Cleveland Clinic. Since it had only been three weeks since Pat was accepted for a heart transplant, it seemed unbelievable to her, and she pondered about getting her heart cut out, not knowing whether she would wake up again.

She finally decided that she had to do this, packed her bag and was ready to leave. Before leaving, Pat told her mother, who was still up, the reason they were leaving at l:30 AM.

They called two of their sons. One daughter-in-law planned to stay with Pat's mother.

Pat went down the hall to pick out a book to read. As she was walking back to the kitchen, her defibrillator kicked in and shocked her. Her heart beat may have been too high. While lying on the floor, Pat had about three more shocks that shook her whole body. Although it wasn't exactly painful, Pat did not want that to happen again. She looked over at poor Charles who was sitting on a chair, and he exclaimed, "Oh, no, now you can't get the heart." He called 911 and the Cleveland Clinic to tell them what had happened. In the meantime, Pat tried to calm down so her heart rate would lower.

After a policeman arrived, the ambulance from Brimfield pulled up. They knew Pat and Charles well by then. They told the couple that they could not transport Pat to Cleveland, only to Akron General Medical Center. While they tried to decide what to do, the policeman suggested calling a helicopter. The ambulance could drive Pat to the Carter Lumber Company, which had a helicopter pad, and was only about two miles from their home. As soon as Pat heard, 'Carter Lumber Company', she knew everything would be okay. A few minutes later, the helicopter arrived from Cleveland. In the meantime, their sons picked up their dad and drove to Cleveland.

Pat had never been on a helicopter ride before, and did not really enjoy it because she could not see out the window. She had wires all over her body while she watched the monitor which seemed to be right in her face. She tried to be composed to keep her heart rate down. Belly breathing helped, and she did a lot of it that night.

The trip took about fifteen minutes, after which Pat was put on a gurney and wheeled through the halls to the elevator, and through more halls to the surgery ward. The trip seemed to take forever. When Pat arrived there, she was amazed to see her husband and two sons already there, and came to the conclusion that they must have driven very fast to get there before she did.

Pat was given an IV and was hooked up to many wires. She felt relaxed, however, and figured she had been given something to quiet her. As she was being rolled into surgery, she asked if the pacemaker-defibrillator would be removed and they confirmed that it would. The last thing Pat remembered was saying a prayer to her Dad in heaven to help her through the surgery. As she was praying, she saw a square opening on top of her with two hands descending. This illusion was probably caused by the medication she was given.

When Pat awakened from the surgery, Pat could see a doctor close by saying, "Remember, don't ever drink or eat grapefruit." Since she was on a ventilator and had been given morphine, Pat could not respond. She felt as though she was rocking on a boat and saw everyone fighting and shooting, an illusion most likely caused by the morphine. She felt rather terrified, but actually was more concerned about gaining ten pounds, which she had heard happens sometimes after surgery.

Pat later learned from her sons that Dr. McCarthy, the head surgeon at the Clinic, performed her surgery at about six AM. They told her that their Dad started shaking and was feeling bad, so they decided to find him a hotel room. Because the Shah of Iran was in Cleveland with an entourage of approximately four hundred with him, he had a whole floor of the clinic to himself. After finding a hotel down by Jacob's Field, Charles went to bed and said he felt better there. The boys went back to the Clinic and waited until the surgery was over at 10:00 AM. They talked to the doctor at 11 AM, and saw their mother later in the day after she awakened. Pat asked them where their Dad was, and they told her that he was so tired earlier, they put him to bed. After a short visit, they left to go back to the hotel room where they found him unconscious on the floor. They dressed him, carried him to the car, and drove him to the Emergency Room at the Cleveland Clinic. After many tests were done, the doctors decided to keep Charles overnight. The boys went back to the hotel room to sleep.

In the meantime, a nurse brought a paper for Pat to sign to try a research drug. Since there was no one there from her family with whom to discuss this, she thought it over for a while, and decided that she should sign the paper in order to help someone else. *After all,* she reasoned, *I was lucky to get a heart, and feel like I should try to help others who might be in my condition.* Pat had been informed that she had to start taking the medication the first day, so she signed the papers, and also other papers to allow the surgeons to use a few extra pieces of her heart when they did biopsies.

When Pat's sons came in to see her the next day, they told her that Charles was in the hospital with a virus and had to stay away from her for ten days. Pat was thankful that he did not have a heart attack or a stroke, which she had envisioned at first. She talked to Charles on the phone, and knew he was all right. Charles was released later on that day.

After the ventilator was taken out, Pat had a very raspy voice. A specialist was called in who put a tube down her throat and told her not to worry. He said her voice should return by itself, but in case it did not, there was a minor surgery which could be done. Pat's voice did come back within a few days.

After Pat arrived in her hospital room, she was in a lot of pain from the opening of the bone in her chest. The heart had no pain because all of the nerves were cut when they replaced her old one. Pat was told to stay flat on her back and not roll either way, and her swollen right foot and ankle was propped up on pillows.

A lovely person, not a nurse, came every morning and night to fix Pat's pillows a certain way under her arms to make her more comfortable and the pain more bearable. People there thought of that person as a saint, for she always helped everyone to feel better.

Pat had an incision on her right side near her collar bone with a blood vein going down to her right breast, which was full of blood and looked almost black. That took six weeks to clear, although at the present time, it is still swollen.

Not being allowed to eat for about six days did not bother Pat, but the second day that she was allowed to eat, she was brought grapefruit juice. Since she had been told not to eat grapefruit or drink grapefruit juice ever again, Pat questioned why they brought her grapefruit juice. It was taken away and replaced by orange juice.

While in the hospital, Pat was told to practice each day taking the nineteen prescriptions that she needed because she would be in charge of taking them once she arrived home.

Three of the medications were for anti-heart rejection and one was a placebo. She was told that one of the anti-rejection medications would make her thighs weak. Besides the other medications, Pat had IV medication twice a day. The total cost of the pills for the first month, not counting the IV medication, was $1,600. The operation cost between $100,000 and $125,000.

A biopsy was done a few days after the surgery which showed rejection, but Pat was told not to worry as it was not an unusual occurrence. She was given Prednisone and other drugs to take five times a day. Because the anti-rejection medicine could cause a low immunity, Pat was told to stay away from live plants, dogs, cats, birds, mold, or anything with germs or spores. The medication also washed out calcium from her body, so she was told to take four extra-strength Tums a day, and later on, Fosamax. Pat's nails broke after three weeks, three of her teeth broke off after six weeks, and she grew a beard.

A charming older woman, who was in Pat's room, watched game shows and every sporting event on her television set, including the Indians and football games. Pat joined her in watching the entertainment, because she did not really feel like reading or doing anything else at the time.

After spending a week in bed, Pat was allowed to walk, which was encouraged in order to gain strength. As she was walking in the hall, inching along with baby steps, a man went whizzing by her with his IV. Pat commented, "You are doing well." He answered, "Keep up the good work," and suddenly Pat realized that she could walk at a near normal pace because she had a new heart in her, even though she did not yet feel emotionally connected to it. She understood that emotions have a lot to do with healing, so decided to accept the heart. She even named the heart 'Suzie', after a bouncy friend who was a lot of fun. Since that time, 'Suzie' and Pat have accomplished many things and have enjoyed life.

The next day, Charles brought Pat a digital blood pressure kit and a thermometer, so that she could take her blood pressure twice a day and her temperature. She was told to start walking on the treadmill every day, at first for ten minutes, and later working up to an hour.

A meeting was held with all the people waiting for a heart, and they happened to be all males. One man had been waiting for five months for a heart, another for four months, and another from Indiana who was there with his wife. Pat tried to tell them what the transplant was like without frightening them too much.

On the ninth day after surgery, Pat was ready to leave for home, but was first given some blood. Four hours later, only one third of the blood had transferred into her body. The doctor was furious because he said the blood was no longer any good, and urged Pat to stay another day for more blood. However, she was anxious to leave.

On the ride home, every bump in the road hurt her chest even though she was taking pain pills. She was so excited to see her Aunt Dorothy and Uncle Clyde waiting in the driveway, she hopped out of the car and danced around.

They seemed amazed to see her moving like that. Pat trotted over to the door and stepped up on the step when her legs collapsed. She then pulled herself up with her arms. Later on, when she bent down to get something out of the bottom of the refrigerator, she could not get up. She crawled to the cupboard and again pulled herself up with her arms. By this time, it was evident to her that she needed to strengthen her legs. Pat was given special exercises for that purpose.

The medicines Pat was taking made food taste terrible. Orange juice tasted like salt water and most sweet foods were not palatable. The only nourishment that tasted good was milk and ice cream. Pat had been told to gain weight, but could hardly eat. Her Aunt Dorothy made her some salt less but tasty tomato rice soup and turkey soup which Pat was able to digest. On one occasion, at eleven o'clock at night, Pat was dreaming of macaroni salad, so her ninety-three year old mother made her some macaroni salad. She only took two bites of it because it did not taste quite right to her, either.

A nurse came twice a day to give Pat an IV of medication and help her with her pills. Pat was so weak that she could not open the bottles, which were childproof, but also adult proof, especially after heart surgery. Charles tried to hook up the IVs, but was unable to because his fingers were too big and his hands shook.

The second week home, they drove to the Cleveland Clinic for another biopsy. Pieces were taken out of Pat's heart and tested for rejection. Waiting until a person has symptoms is too late. They called the next day and told Pat that the report was I-A, which was very slight. They kept her on the same medicine.

While on the way to the Cleveland clinic, Pat told Charles how lucky she was to have him because he had worked so hard at Ford Motor Company for thirty seven years and they had wonderful benefits which enabled her to receive a new heart.

The very next week, Pat's brother, Jerry, was in town for a school reunion. He accompanied Charles and Pat to Cleveland for another biopsy. They arrived home at suppertime after a long day at the hospital. Pat's mother had prepared a nice dinner for all of them.

Pat was resting on the couch when she heard a loud crash in the bathroom. She tried to open the door, but it would not open. She called out to her husband, but he did not answer. Jerry, who was downstairs, ran up and pried the door open. Charles' head was squeezed in the door, and, as he came to, he asked for a pillow to rest there for a couple of hours. Suddenly, he asked for help to get to the toilet where he threw up and choked, while his eyes were rolling around. Pat called 911. When they ambulance arrived and the paramedics found no pulse, they quickly lifted Charles on the stretcher and hurried out the door. Pat called their son to meet his Dad at the hospital, while Jerry followed him in the ambulance. Pat stayed home and prayed.

The next afternoon, Charles' doctor called the family to come in, and Pat went to the hospital in a wheelchair and wearing a mask. A nurse whom they knew explained the situation and told them that Charles might not live through the night. Although Pat was shocked and upset, she told the doctor they had signed power of attorney and living wills, and that she wanted him to have the best care possible because they had good insurance coverage. Although the nurse in ICU did not want Pat to be with Charles because of all the germs, Dr. Maxwell did let her go in for five minutes.

Charles was able to tell Pat that Father Lyons had given him the sacrament of the sick. Pat told Charles that she loved him and that he was a wonderful husband and father. She told him, "Don't worry, don't be afraid." Charles was bleeding internally while they gave him blood. The doctor cauterized the spot and performed surgery. All of their sons and extended family came to see Charles. A nurse finally called Pat and told her to stop people from coming there since Charles was liable to pick up some germs. Charles did well for a few days. One of his sons and his wife stayed with him. Their fourth son, who lived in California, came to see him and then returned to California.

Charles took a turn for the worse and was put on a ventilator. Pat played a recording of their new grandson, Peter, gooing and gurgling, for Charles. Charles tried to respond after he heard it, but was unable to talk. After being on the ventilator for two weeks, the doctors wanted to take him off. Pat begged them to keep him on the ventilator until their son from California could get there. Everyone said goodbye to Charles and told them they loved him. The doctor gave him a shot and turned off the ventilator. He took three breaths on his own and he was gone. The family talked to the doctor and asked for an autopsy because Charles' brother had just passed away similarly and they wanted to know what kind of inherited disease he had that might be passed on to his sons.

The funeral was beautiful. Their priest, Father Lyons, and their pastor, Father McGovern, helped and supported Pat and her family through all their illnesses and the funeral. Pat was surprised by the many people who came to the funeral. Charles had been a football, basketball and baseball player, coach, and sports fan. Many of the three hundred people who came were from the teams Charles had coached or with whom he had played. Charles had a way with kids, and youngsters had always flocked to him. Toddlers sat on his lap who would not even go to their own relatives. Charles treated them with M&Ms or a stick of gum. At the graveside, some of the great nieces put packs of M&Ms on his casket. Charles, Pat's loving husband, was sixty six years old when he passed away.

Pat belonged to HMO Health Ohio. When she received her new heart, she was sixty four years old, not yet on Medicare. HMO paid for all the expenses of her heart, the hospitalization, pacemaker and defibrillator, surgery, Charles' hospitalization, and medical bills which were over $300,000. All Pat had to pay was $9.00. She was grateful for that, and still praises HMO.

Jerry stayed for six weeks after the funeral and drove Pat everywhere and helped her in many ways. Pat was overwhelmed taking care of an estate, since she was still recovering, still hurting and on pain pills. During that time, the sewer system also kept backing up. She appreciated all that Jerry did for her.

Pat also had a lot of support from other family, cousins, and good friends. People brought food. One friend in particular, Barbara, still visits her every week.

After the first month, Pat had biopsies every two weeks, and was obliged to have blood work done in between at Akron General Medical Center. Because of the funeral, she delayed having a regular catheterization done until the eighth week. Her friend, Aggie, took her at five AM for the procedure which showed a clogged artery in the new heart. Pat was filled with grief and disappointment. After deliberating, an angioplasty was performed right away, and a stent inserted. She stayed at the hospital overnight. Her rejection level was consistently 1-A or 1-B which required no extra medication.

Pat's chest bone hurt, especially when she drove the car, and she was not allowed take a pain pill when she drove. She complained to the doctors who thought she may have had inflammation of the bone. The condition cleared up after two more weeks of proper medication. Pat lost about ten pounds during this time.

Unfortunately, because of the Prednisone, Pat started growing facial hair, thick eyebrows and hair. Although her hair was supposed to turn dark, that did not happen.

Pat was in the hospital once again the day before Thanksgiving with diverticulitis. She blamed her difficulty of focusing on things to grief, surgery recovery, and being on the heart-lung machine which she had heard could give people cognitive problems. The holiday season that year was quiet, and rather sad, except for the joy her grandchildren and the rest of the family brought her. She was happy to learn that she was going to have two new grandbabies.

The first week of a bitter cold January, as Pat walked to the mail box, she realized she did it with no heart pain. She felt that she was on the mend. She also drove to the doctor's office. The doctors decided that her immunity was too low, so she was given some kind of gamma globulin IV for two months. It took four hours each month while they checked her blood pressure and temperature. Pat was also given a sulfa drug which she took for about a year to protect her from infections.

Even though she still had biopsies every month, by spring of 2000 she felt as though she was thirty five again. She could walk at her own speed, and her medications were reduced in strength. She had no viruses or colds and her chest pain was completely gone even when she coughed. She felt more like her normal self because she had the heart transplant. Pat actually felt well enough to paint the basement walls and floor at a reasonable pace and spent most of the winter accomplishing that task.

Of course, there were still some problems. Pat was required to have catheterizations for the rest of her life because the medication she was taking could cause clogged arteries, diabetes, glaucoma, skin cancer, and many other ailments. She had cataract surgery in the fall of 2000 because she could not see the green lights when driving. That was probably hurried along by the medicine.

Pat still had swelling of her ankles, especially the right ankle. Although it did not bother her when walking, she thought that it made her look terrible. Before that, at Christmas in 1999, the swelling had gone up her right side into her right breast, and her right arm and hand. She had tests done, and was told that about ten percent of heart transplant patients experienced swelling in the feet. The doctors did not know what caused her right foot to swell to such a degree. The swelling in her arm and hand disappeared in about a month, supposedly because it had something to do with her lymph glands.

In the year 2001, Pat contracted a bad infection and landed in the Cleveland Clinic once again. The doctors thought they would discover the cause of the infection but never did. She was given Azithromycin and Cipro through an IV which burned like fire.

Pat was in the hospital for nine days, and roomed with a very feisty lady named Jane who was an architect. Jane told Pat that she was so ill when she arrived there, she couldn't walk up the stairs without help. She was put on the heart transplant list and was waiting for a new heart.

Pat's son, who was in town to stay with his grandmother, visited his mother in the hospital. While visiting, the three of them started conversing about the Cleveland Indians, and ultimately Jane and Pat's son were involved in a heated argument. Pat reprimanded her son for upsetting Jane since she was so ill, but noticed that they both seemed to enjoy arguing.

Jane was given special medication by IV and was watched closely. Pat thought that it was amazing to see how the medication worked, because Jane got up and took off with her IV pole. Jane took Pat with her to a Mass on Sunday which was two buildings away, and she trotted right over. She also used a treadmill, went to the lobby to read a paper, and wore Pat out. Pat had not experienced anything like that, but she and Jane got along famously and enjoyed each other's company. Pat asked Jane to ask her doctor how long a heart transplant would last, and the doctor said probably ten years. He told them a story of the first transplanted heart patient who was still living, smoking, drinking and stealing cars. Jane said she would not have trouble learning to smoke and drink but she would need lessons on stealing cars. They all laughed.

After Pat left the hospital, she found out that Jane's heart transplant was performed a few days afterwards. Another woman from England who had been waiting for seven months also had her heart transplant.

For the next two years, Pat felt better. She still had the biopsies every three months with zero rejection. She was sent to a kidney specialist, Dr. Boshkos, who tested her kidneys and found out she had about 30% kidney function and concluded that it was permanent damage from the Neoral drug. He wanted Pat to take a kidney friendly drug, but the Cleveland Clinic refused because they had no experience with that particular drug.

On March 6, 2003, Pat fell on ice in the cemetery and broke her shoulder. It was a traumatic time for her, because she kept re-injuring her shoulder which she had assumed would heal in about two months. However, it took her all summer before she was free of pain and could once again sleep well. Pat was behind in all her projects. When she saw Dr. Boshkos again, he did more tests and found out that Pat's kidney function was going lower and suggested dialysis. He also wrote again to Dr. Starling at the Heart Transplant Medicine Dept. Dr. Starling sent Pat to a kidney specialist at the Cleveland Clinic for a consultation. The kidney specialist ordered a special kidney test on September 2 at Robinson Memorial Hospital in Ravenna.

In June, Pat's cousin took her to the Cleveland Clinic again for some special blood work for the research drug she had been taking called RAD. While they waited to be seen, they met thirteen other people who had heart transplants, two women and eleven men. Most were middle aged to about seventy, but one man was probably in his twenties and one woman in her thirties—she had two children. Some of the heart transplants were from Michigan, New York, and Indiana, and one was from Cleveland. Pat asked them if they had kidney problems and none of them did. They all looked very healthy and active except one who had developed cancer and was in a wheelchair. Pat checked to see if any of them had a swollen foot, but did not see any.

In August, Dr. Starling's office called to put Pat on a new drug, Cellcept, while gradually reducing the Neoral. Two weeks later, Pat developed diarrhea, which was a common side effect. They told her that her body would get used to Cellcept. Pat took Immodium, but by the third week, was getting sicker and sicker.

On Labor Day weekend, she went to Akron General Medical Center because she was very dizzy. After waiting for five hours and watching five helicopter landings, Pat started to feel better. She went home after midnight. The next morning, her son took her back to the hospital where they gave her an IV because she was dehydrated, along with some strong medication. They went back home afterwards.

On Tuesday after Labor Day, Pat's cousin, Bonnie, took her to the Ravenna hospital for the kidney test. Upon arriving home, she called the Cleveland Clinic. Dr. Starling's office and his nurse practitioner told her to go directly to Cleveland Clinic Emergency Room. After calling her primary doctor and getting a referral, Pat's son took her to the ER. For two days, Pat was given tests to make sure she did not have any other kidney disease, was given IVs, and was taken off Cellcept and put on Imuran. The difference in the price was considerable. Cellcept had cost $840 a month, while Imuran cost only $5.00 a month.

Pat had had no rejections for two years, but after another biopsy, had a moderate rejection, which was most likely caused by losing fluids from diarrhea. The medicines were increased, and biopsies were performed in October and November which showed moderate rejection and nodules on Pat's lungs. On December 22, Pat had zero rejection and was very relieved to have the good news before Christmas. She had had enough bad news in the past year, 2003, including a death in the family. Pat's Mother had a pacemaker installed, and her beloved sister-in-law, Grace, passed away.

Pat experienced a humorous incident in November when she and her mother were at a wedding at Tangier Restaurant. They went to the Ladies' Room and noticed a woman whom Pat thought resembled her cousin's wife's sister. Pat asked her if she was the sister who had a liver transplant, but she said that she was not, although she was the one who had a stroke. However, the sister with the liver transplant was at the wedding. At that moment, a woman came out of a stall and said, "Well, I had a bone marrow transplant." Everyone laughed. Ladies' Room conversations used to be about children, trips, aches and pains, but in the future everyone will probably be talking about their transplants.

When Pat was having her November biopsy, she noticed two men who were in their seventies who had just received new hearts. One man, who had his heart transplant for two weeks, and the other man who had his heart transplant for one month, were walking around like nothing had ever happened. Pat asked the latter if he had any pain and he said that he didn't. It made Pat feel like she was the hospital baby because she needed a barrel of Novocaine to numb her skin, and squirmed and jumped when they took pieces from her heart. She was told that, if she had no more trouble, she should only have two more biopsies and then none after the fifth year. However, she will still have to have a catheterization once a year for the rest of her life.

Pat is looking forward to spring of 2004, is thankful for every day, and prays often for her donor. She urges everyone who reads this story to please sign your name on your driver's license as an organ donor, and urge friends and family to do the same. It's a good idea to discuss this with your family so that they will know your wishes if something should happen, because sometimes it is a difficult decision for a family to make. Older people who have died, who were in good health otherwise before their death, may also donate their hearts for others their age. What a wonderful gift it would be for someone who needs a heart like Pat did!

Pat wrote a poem which follows:

A MEDICAL MIRACLE
Patricia Albanese

My nickname has always been Pat
I wear purple dresses with a red had.
Oh, yes, I am young at heart
But the rest of me is falling apart.
I had a transplant four years ago,
It made me a new person, that I know.
I take lots of medicine, that's for sure
And eat lots of vegetables, fruits, all salt less and pure.
Five times a day I take all my pills,
Stay away from people with sickness and ills.
My immunity is low, must keep this heart good,
I have to behave, I know I should.
A special gift from a family so bold,
That person's in heaven, so I've been told.
The reason for this poem, you see,
Is to be a donor for someone like me.

ED MITCHELL'S REMARKABLE RECOVERY

Edward Eugene Mitchell, a calm, quiet-spoken, and respectable man, had driven a semi-trailer truck long distance for forty-two years before retiring in the year 2000. During the years he was driving, he was away from home much of the time, but his occupation enabled him to adequately support his wife, Peg, and their three children. He really enjoyed driving, and did not even mind sleeping in the truck. However, Ed's diet consisted mostly of greasy fried foods at truck stops while on the road, which he ate as a matter of course. He never worried about the effect of fatty foods on his cholesterol. Ed did not even know what his cholesterol was at that time for he never had his blood taken. During some of the forty-two years Ed drove the semi, no one was aware of how dangerous it was to eat fatty foods.

Of course, when Ed was home, Peg, his wife of forty-eight years, cooked delicious meals of chicken, turkey, fish, and occasional beef roasts, along with vegetables and fruit.

One day while Ed was delivering freight in Oklahoma City, in the summer of 1998, he felt some pain in his chest and thought it was perhaps an upset stomach or a hiatal hernia, so he called Peg to tell her of his distress. She immediately called the heart specialist. The specialist scheduled an angiogram (catheterization) for Ed the next day. It was discovered that Ed had five blockages in his arteries, three of which were over forty percent. An angioplasty was performed and stents were installed in two of the arteries with blockages. In the third artery, what they called a roto-rooter was installed. The doctor decided not to do anything about the two smaller than forty percent blockages because he suspected that the small veins might rupture.

Ed felt fine immediately and went back to work driving the semi shortly after the angioplasty. After he retired from his job in the year 2000, he went regularly to his family doctor who told him he was doing fine.

Ed, being a very active person, was not entirely satisfied with staying home, so he obtained a part time job driving a postal truck. He delivered mail early in the morning and later in the afternoon, and was enjoying life.

At about 11:30 AM on July 15, 2004, while Ed was outside working in the yard, he felt some pressure in his chest, but no pain anywhere else. Peg was visiting her sister, Hazel, who was having tests at Albemarle Hospital in Elizabeth City, North Carolina, seventeen miles from Barco, where Ed and Peg lived. Ed called Peg, who got in touch with the heart specialist at Albemarle, to arrange for tests for Ed. Peg drove home immediately, called her other sister, Irene, to meet them at the emergency room at Albemarle. Since it took twenty minutes to half an hour to get to and from the hospital, Ed and Peg thought it would be best for her to drive Ed there, especially since there was no cardiovascular ambulance in Barco. Dr. White later told Peg that Ed would have been gone in another twenty minutes, so they definitely made the right decision.

They arrived at 1:30 PM at Emergency, where a catheterization determined that Ed needed to have a quadruple heart bypass. Ed was immediately transferred by cardiovascular ambulance to Sentera Hospital in Norfolk, Virginia. The quadruple heart bypass was done at eight AM on July 16, 2004.

Ed was in the recovery room at 1:45 PM, and at first he did not realize there was a tube in his throat, but was told that he had tried to pull it out. He had three veins taken out of his right leg, and one out of his left leg, but had no trouble at all with the incisions. While in the hospital, like all heart patients, he was given a Mended Hearts Pillow. Ed was sent home in four days, and took his pillow with him. All of the heart patients there had signed his pillow.

Ed was fortunate because he was able to get out of bed by himself, and started walking up and down the driveway the day he arrived home. Of course, he felt some discomfort because he had to learn to sleep on his back. Ed had formerly always slept on his stomach, and it takes a while to get used to sleeping on one's back. Ed decided to sleep on the couch because it was easier for him to get up from the couch than from his bed. He only noticed one thing that he questioned, and it was an overlapping of the skin on his upper neck, but that righted itself in time.

Ed kept busy the first month doing puzzles. He and Peg belonged to a catalog club which charged only $2.00 for different puzzle scenes which usually cost $29 in a retail store. Ed mounted them on paper and framed them, and now has a nice collection on his wall, like a colorful art museum.

After one month, Ed felt like his old self, and was even allowed to drive, which was a great relief to him. Sitting in the back seat of the car with Peg as his chauffeur was not his idea (or hers) of having fun during that month.

In August, just one week after Ed started to drive again, Peg felt some pain in her chest. Ed drove her to the hospital, where she had an angiogram. They were delighted to find out afterwards that she had no blockages.

Ed started the physical therapy and enjoyed using all the machines. On September 19, he and Peg decided to drive to Akron, Ohio, where their son and daughter lived. Ed drove the whole distance without any problem. The family enjoyed being together for their great grandson's second birthday party, and a family reunion.

Today Ed looks and feels great. His 192 pounds is just right for his six feet frame. All he has to do different now is take heart medication, cholesterol medication, blood pressure medication, and an aspirin a day. Peg changed her method of cooking just a little. She no longer uses salt, but instead uses a salt substitute. Life is back to normal for both of them.

On October 4, 2004, Ed started to work on his mail run again. He is thankful for all the excellent medical care he received, and that he recovered so quickly.

JERRY BEAN'S MIRACLES

Jerry Bean was a successful business man who lived in California. He knew every mathematical concept for running his financial enterprise. In 1990, Jerry had one of the most successful years in his entire life. His family was fine, emotionally and financially. His company was doing great, and he and his wife, Leanna, were looking forward with anticipation to the birth of their first grandchild on December 12. However, something happened on December 11, 1990, that was to alter their lives. Jerry developed an aneurysm on his upper aorta, the main artery coming out of his heart, which subsequently traveled from his heart into his left leg. Jerry's aorta had burst inwardly (a dissected aorta). He was taken to Kaiser-Permanente Hospital and it was decided to life fly him to a well known Stanford Medical Center in Palo Alto. Since the weather was too foggy to fly, he was taken there in an ambulance. Statistics show that ninety percent of people with a dissected aorta die before surgery and do not live through this condition, so Jerry was considered one of the lucky ones. He viewed his recovery as a true miracle. His surgery cost over $257,000, but his co-pay was only $5.00. Jerry's surgery took about five hours. He was heavily medicated, and started bleeding inside. One of the stitches broke open and the blood was sucked out. Jerry went into cardiac arrest. Jerry does not remember much of anything during his stay in the hospitals, a total of three different hospitals.

When he looked in his wallet, he had a fishing license but did not remember ever fishing. Jerry did not remember flying, and subsequently lost his pilot's license. He did not remember having his wedding ring remade. Because his life had always seemed complicated in many ways, it did not surprise him when he later learned that he had had transfusions of fifty three pints of blood and $25,000 worth of drugs during the coma he experienced for four weeks after December 11. In January, 1991, the doctors explained to Leanna that it might be time to pull the plug and give less aggressive care because Jerry had been brain dead for one full month. The priest was called in, and explained the Church's position on the extension of a hopeless life, consequently Jerry was given the Last Rites. Leanna stayed at Jerry's bedside at the hospital, along with the rest of his family and friends in California. Everyone from the church and school prayed for him, and helped him through this crisis. Father Wilkimey anointed Jerry with holy water he brought home from Lourdes. Jerry's family from Ohio was called to California. His sister and eighty-four year old mother brought a medal with them which they had received from Medjugorje, Yugoslavia. His mother rubbed it on his limbs, head and heart, saying, "I am Mother Bean and I want you to wake up and talk to me. Do you hear me, Jerry?" Jerry woke up enough to say, "Hello, Mother Bean," although he had never called her that before. The nurses were summoned to witness his awakening. One of the nurses said, "If you hear my voice, squeeze my hand." Jerry did squeeze her hand. He considered this the second miracle. Jerry went back to sleep. When Leanna arrived at the hospital, she was disappointed when she tried talking to her husband and did not get a response. Their daughter delivered the baby a day after Jerry's catheterization procedure.

He awakened, but they did not know if he would be okay or a vegetable. He had a valve attached to his throat to help him talk when someone pushed the valve. His first words were, "Get mother a chair" in a muffled voice. His mother kept repeating, "Jerry, you had a stroke, but you are going to be fine." It was a good sign when Jerry said, after hearing that phrase constantly, "Quit telling me that!"

Jerry prayed to God that he would live to see his grandchild baptized, and he was there when Bucky was baptized, through the manipulation of the priest. Jerry greatly appreciated his intervention. Jerry was in the hospital a total of three and a half months with serious complications from the lack of blood to his brain and spine. He had lost all mathematical knowledge, even adding and subtracting, which frightened him immensely. Jerry started to pray the Rosary to help regain his mental capacities.

One morning a few days later, Leanna called him with a fairly complex business problem, and he literally shouted out the answer. From that day on, his mind responded to math. His walking gait gradually improved. Both are right hemisphere functions, and Jerry considered that another miracle. After Jerry returned home, he had so much support. There were people who sent daily meals while the whole family was under extreme stress. They were some of the same people of his parish whose constant prayers and cards helped him recover. He felt thankful that people took over his volunteer duties at his church, too.

Jerry's mother and his sister, Pat, stayed at Jerry and Leanna's house for ten days. There were as many as twenty-one people coming and going and helping with the housework during the time Jerry was in the hospital. After Jerry was taken off the ventilator, he still felt very tired. However, after therapy was started, it seemed like no time at all that he was sitting on the side of his bed. Once he started to feed himself, even though it looked robotic, Pat and his mother left for Ohio. Pat's husband stayed longer to take Jerry to his doctor appointments. Jerry was sent to a nursing home in Saratoga, California, for seven weeks, after which he went to rehab at Kaiser Rehabilitation in Vallej. He came home just before his birthday in March. His improvement was steady, his coordination improved, and he was determined to drive the car, which he did. Jerry had a hard time getting up from the bed and couch, so he used forearm canes. In about seven weeks, he was able to walk around the block.

He started looking forward to eating more food since he had lost so much weight. Jerry did have one setback, however. He went to a neighbor's wedding in May and felt like he was ready to dance, play and keep up with the crowd. He made it home from the wedding just fifteen minutes before a mild heart attack got his immediate attention. The message to slow down came through strong and clear. He asked the doctor, 'How long do you think I will live?" The doctor replied, "At least eight years." Jerry was in the hospital for a week. After arriving home, he started to drive again, and slowly returned to almost normal, although he still became easily tired.

Katie, his youngest daughter, who was in the third grade, worried every day whether her dad would remember to pick her up after school, because he had forgotten to do that a couple of times. Although Jerry to this day is still considered disabled, he can function as well as most retired people.

DORIS IRVINE'S TRAUMA

Doris Irvine was born in Sharon, Pennsylvania, on July 26, 1927. She was a healthy child, teen and young adult. In 1944, she married Al Irvine and they had two children; one daughter, Leslee, and one son, Bob.

Doris kept busy taking care of her family, and had many other interests. When she was in her thirties, her doctor found out that she had high blood pressure, and prescribed medication to keep it under control.

Doris' husband, Al, passed away in 1982 while they lived in Kentucky. He had worked at Goodyear Tire & Rubber Company as an engineer for many years and during that time, the family lived in several different states.

Doris decided to move back to Stow, Ohio, where she bought a condo. She started doing water exercises at the Cuyahoga Falls Natatorium where she met Dick Moorehead. They were married in 1986.

When Doris turned seventy-three years old, she went to her family doctor's office for a routine exam. She had a stress test, and after that a catheterization at City Hospital which showed that she had five blockages of eighty five to ninety percent. Stents could not be used because of the unusual ninety-three degree angle of her arteries. Bypass heart surgery was performed, and, instead of coming home in five days, Doris actually spent six weeks in the hospital.

After the surgery, Doris did well immediately, and was moved to step-down. While there, she was eating yogurt when she felt a slight pain in her chest. The nurse, who was a friend of her daughter's, gave Doris nitroglycerine every five minutes. The next thing she knew was that they moved her back to the cardiac unit since she was having a heart attack. Doris developed three different types of pneumonia, and had much difficulty breathing. She was moved to ICU where she was heavily sedated and on a ventilator.

At that time, Doris was distraught and told her daughter she wanted to die. Leslee reassured Doris that she would return to good health, for Leslee had worked in the cardiac unit since she became a nurse, and had seen about everything that could happen. Doris' husband, Dick, was very supportive.

Doris was moved to Semper Care and thought her doctors were very comforting, except for one who came in at six AM every morning with a little too much enthusiasm. Other than that, she had super care in ICU for two weeks, and Semper Care for four weeks. At one point in ICU, she opened her eyes and noticed her son and daughter-in-law from Cleveland walking down the hall, and she thought, "This is it, they have called my family in." Her daughter, of course, could drop in anytime. Doris slept a lot in ICU because of sedation, and does not remember everything that occurred.

Once off the ventilator, Doris had many breathing problems, possibly because she had smoked for forty years. However, she had quit smoking fifteen years before the surgery.

Doris was very apprehensive when she was in Semper care, and could not seem to sleep. She begged for a sleeping pill, but was not given any because they told her that it affects sleep REM. Three weeks of feeling anxiety and deep trouble could have been relieved by a non-addictive sleep aid.

All of her doctors, however, were very kind and reassuring. When she was in ICU, one pretty young social worker was especially kind. The doctors brought resident doctors with them to observe her and she was surrounded many times by medical personnel. Doris, of course, was in a fog some of the time that this parade of doctors and others came and passed.

Doris was finally released from the hospital in the middle of March, and was extremely glad to be home. She was very weak and used a walker. Dick helped the home care therapist, and used a baby monitor in the master bedroom while he slept in the guest room.

Doris' eldest granddaughter, Kirsten, an occupational therapist, and her two boys from Indiana, drove to see her while she was in ICU, but Doris could not talk at that time. Kirsten stayed in Doris' condo while in Ohio.

On Doris' seventy-fifth birthday, Kirsten planned a party with sixty people in attendance at Silver Lake Towers party room. Leslee bought red roses and gave a rose to Doris while she told a story about her. Kirsten's husband, Wally, sang a song.

After six weeks of rehabilitation, and thirty-six sessions at Cuyahoga Falls General Hospital, Doris was able to walk without the walker. While all the trauma was happening, people from the Episcopal church came to see her and prayed for her. She received at least one hundred cards.

Doris is now taking her medication, sees her family doctor and cardiologist and is doing everything necessary for a quality life. She is also going to water exercise again and does needlework in her spare time.

GLORIA'S STORY—ON THE BRINK OF A HEART ATTACK

Gloria Pimentel was born in Guadalajara, in the state of Jalisco, in the southern part of Mexico. She grew up in a middle class environment. After she and her husband married, he took her to Tijuana, where she was shocked to see the dire poverty which existed in that part of Mexico so close to the United States. She felt that she had been spoiled as a child. Besides raising her family, she has tried to help others ever since.

Gloria was in reasonably good health until about six years ago, when she suddenly felt weak and slightly dizzy as she was driving along the freeway on her way to work. Her ears began to ring. She panicked, and drove off the freeway ramp to see her doctor who was located about a mile away. As soon as she told him how weird she was feeling, he connected her to the EKG machine. It showed that everything was normal, and there was no sign of heart problems. His diagnosis was that she had a panic attack, and that she was now fine.

A year after that episode, she started having problems with a rise in her blood pressure. Her doctor put her on medication for one month and it brought her blood pressure down to normal. However, she complained to the doctor about the constant diarrhea she was experiencing, so he took her off the medication. Gloria's blood pressure stayed normal for two years. Her doctor, whom she had been seeing for twenty years, died suddenly of a massive heart attack. She felt totally lost, for she relied on him and his expertise.

Gloria's insurance company placed her with another doctor with whom she set up an appointment. She told the doctor that she had been feeling lethargic, had no energy, and sometimes felt like her heart was skipping beats. While giving Gloria a physical check up, the doctor discovered that Gloria's blood pressure was rather high. She put Gloria on medication, which made her very ill. Gloria had diarrhea, a splitting headache, a dry mouth, and she could not breathe comfortably while climbing stairs. Her heart began to skip and she felt like she was about to drop dead. Her legs, arms, and hands were bloated to three times their normal size due to Edema.

Gloria complained about her terrible reactions to the medication, but the doctor insisted that her body had to get used to it. However, Gloria ended up in the hospital at the brink of a heart attack. A heart specialist was called in and he ordered all kinds of tests, including an angiogram, but nothing showed up. He and another cardiologist could find nothing wrong with Gloria's heart. She overheard them talking. One said to the other, "I don't understand, she had all the symptoms. It was only a fraction of a second before she'd have a heart attack—you saw the reports." The other cardiologist scratched his head and replied, "I don't understand it, either."

After five days in the hospital, Gloria was told that she had a very strong heart and it was most likely a heart spasm that caused the symptoms. Gloria was released, and her blood pressure medicine was changed. She was told to monitor the effects closely. Very soon she started to feel the same bad effects, like she was going to drop dead any minute.

She fell on her knees, prayed, and asked God to give her the courage to face the end if it was her time. She prayed that He would give her enough time to put her affairs in order, which she then did. She also prayed that, if it was not her time, to please open a door for her to find a path to healing.

At approximately the same time, Gloria's husband who was ill, refused to have some tests which his doctor suggested. The doctor threw up his arms and asked him, "Do you believe in alternative medicine? Do you want to try natural methods? I simply do not know what else to do with you!"

Gloria's husband jumped at the opportunity and asked to be put in natural healing therapy. Since regular food could never give the body the extraordinary amounts of nutrients it needs to heal, he started a nutritional program based on products made from herbs, veggies, fruits, fruit grains and herbs. These nutrients were highly concentrated in powder, liquid or capsule form. His health quickly improved even to the point where the infection in his leg was healing.

Gloria decided to try the same therapy. When the herbalist/iridologist saw her, she looked into her eyes and told her, "You seem to have serious problems with your circulatory system and your iris shows the beginning of arteriosclerosis. She explained to Gloria that her arteries were clogging and perhaps what she felt was her heart working too hard pumping blood to her lungs and brain.

Gloria acted surprised by the diagnosis, for she had just been given a good bill of health. The herbalist smiled and explained to her that when there are no immediate obstructions in the arteries, doctors do not go beyond that point. Once they see with their machines that blood is running free through the arteries, they are satisfied. She also told Gloria that she had a sodium ring which was the most dangerous kind. Gloria did not doubt her word, for Gloria was a salt-shaker happy-go-lucky kind of girl. She started on the nutritional program and began studying iridology. She was able to read her own eyes as she followed her own healing path. The first symptom which stopped was her heart skipping beats and she could breathe freely again. As if by magic, the pain in her shoulder and upper back disappeared, and her energy returned.

Gloria has been following the nutritional program for over two years. She also graduated from the training program and became a nutritional specialist with herbalist certification.

Since Gloria and her husband discovered that they were both killing themselves with food, they now carefully watch what they eat. They lost a lot of weight. Gloria exercises and is trying to get her husband to exercise with her.

Her blood pressure is normal and she prays that she will never have to take the high blood pressure medication ever again.

To Gloria, it seems like a miracle that has returned to good health and her blood pressure is under control without using chemical drugs. She thanks God every day for helping her discover a new method of living.

MEGAN'S STORY—'ONLY' IS A FOUR-LETTER WORD

After dating almost seven years, Julie and Dan were married on December 3, 1988. They both wanted to have children and started planning their family shortly after their marriage.

However, months, then years, went by with no success. Julie decided to see her doctor, who sent her to an infertility specialist. The specialist prescribed several different medications and performed many different procedures, but nothing seemed to work. Julie felt depressed and guilty. The specialist decided surgery was the next step, and he performed a laparoscope and a D & C in March of 1991. He told Julie that that she had severe endometriosis, but he removed it with a laser. He said that she should feel much better, and he told her that the pain and cramping she felt every month should disappear.

Nevertheless, two weeks later, Julie was in excruciating pain. She called the specialist's office, and the nurse told her to come in immediately. After Julie arrived, she was told that she would have to undergo a pregnancy test before they could give her any medication. Julie agreed to the test, but personally felt that it was a waste of time and money. To her surprise, two minutes later when the nurses returned to her room, they told Julie that she WAS pregnant. They all started to cry after hearing the joyous news.

The first thing Julie did was begin a journal to her baby. The entries will be verbatim.

April 5, 1991

Today is the day Mommy found out she was going to have you. It's one of the happiest days of my life! It took Mommy almost two years to get pregnant with you and I am very excited. When I found out, I cried with the nurses. We are all so happy! I went to the mall and bought baby clothes and pink and blue balloons to decorate so we could tell Daddy. Mommy also bought an "I love my Daddy' bib and placed the positive pregnancy test on it. I decorated the bathroom with everything but confetti and closed the door. Daddy came home and I met him at the front door crying, pretending I had started my period (you will learn about this later in life) and after consoling me for a minute, he went to the bathroom to get me a tissue and saw his surprise. He hollered with joy and spun around into my open arms. He grabbed me, hugged me and we both cried with joy, praising God. WE LOVE YOU!!!!"

Julie had no problems during her pregnancy, and on December 10, 1991, Megan Nichole was born. Julie and Dan were elated with their 'perfect' little girl, who grew at a normal pace. Megan's doctor heard a 'benign' murmur, but saw no cause for concern. Julie noticed that the hair on the back of Megan's neck was always wet with sweat, and mentioned this fact to Dan. Dan remarked, "Don't worry, she's just hot blooded like me."

On October 15, 1993, Julie took Megan to a new doctor for her early two-year checkup. The doctor took an unusually long time listening to Megan's heart. Although she used comforting words and tones, she relayed the rather devastating news that she was not sure that the benign murmur Megan's former doctor had heard was really benign.

Julie immediately made an appointment for Megan for a month later with a pediatric cardiologist who was the only one on their insurance company's list. The month passed slowly at a snail's pace, and seemed to Dan and Julie the longest month they had ever lived. When they finally met the doctor, they did not like his bedside manner, but needed his expertise to help Megan, so were willing to put up with just about anything. He administered an EKG, and told them a plethora of possible, very serious, diagnoses, but said not to worry. He needed a week to study the EKG and would relay the results to them when they returned for another visit.

When they returned to the pediatric cardiologist's office, he asked them, "What did I tell you last time?" Dan and Julie read their notes, to which he replied, "Oh, no, it is much worse than that." Julie felt too frightened to listen, but Dan heard the doctor say that Megan would need open heart surgery by the time she turned five years old. He added, "Go home, don't worry, treat her normal." That was easier said than done. With the power of the scared mother, Julie broke through the bureaucracy of the insurance company which allowed them to go 'off plan' for a second opinion.

After they met Dr. J. at Akron Children's Hospital cardiology department, they knew they were in the right place and felt at ease. He listened to Megan's heart and told them immediately that he could hear the murmur and also added a long list of other defects which they had been told did not exist. He performed an echocardiogram and showed them exactly where the defect was and told them that it was called an Atrial Septal Defect (ASD), which meant that it was a hole in the wall between the two chambers of Megan's heart. Dr. J. explained that her two year old heart was the size of her fist, and the hole was the size of a dime. He added that surgery was needed to repair the hole with a Gortex patch.

The thought of their baby girl having open heart surgery was difficult to accept, they were glad Dr. J told them that he felt there was no point in waiting until Megan was five.

His nurses listened and spoke caringly, saying that they were not just doing their job, but they were allowing God to work through them. They also told Dan and Julie of a congenital heart defect (CHD) support group to which they belonged called HEALING HEARTS. However, the parents were not in the mood to sit around in a circle and cry. They planned to research and prepare for what came next, perhaps by consulting a website or by reading books.

The nurses patiently explained that HEALING HEARTS parent-mentoring program always proved to be a great conduit for some of the best type of information one can find.

HEALING HEARTS specializes in 'been there' knowledge, empathy, support, sharing encouragement and education. Julie was given a telephone number to call. After she called Tammi, a parent mentor, Tammi lovingly devoted many hours of her busy life to answer Julie's questions. Tammi invited Dan and Julie to a HEALING HEARTS meeting where parents of children in all stages of CHD repair began by introducing themselves. When Dan and Julie explained that their daughter had just been diagnosed with ASD, one of the mothers responded with "Oh, only an ASD." They wondered how anyone could use the word 'only' when describing a defect which was going to force their child's chest to be split open and her heart stopped. It took but a few months for them to understand.

Since Dr. J. suspected that it would be hard for Megan's parents to take the next step to make an appointment with a surgeon, he made it for them. He called and told them that the appointment was with Dr. M. at Cleveland Clinic Children's Hospital. After meeting Dr. M., Dan and Julie were convinced that his hands were best for the job, even though they were still somewhat fearful.

February 8, 1994

Dear Megan,

So much is happening and it is hard for mom to deal with all of it. 1st learning of your heart defect and then trying to cope with why my baby? I'm trying to learn as much as I can and to prepare you and me for surgery. I love you so very much and I'm sorry this is happening to you. We have a strong family and we will get through it with that love and the help of God.

May 4, 1994

Dearest Meg,

Today was not an easy day for me. It seemed like everything just caught up with me and I could not take it any longer. So I cried and cried.... I am so glad you were born I look at you and you make me so very happy. I'm sorry you have to go through what you do but mommy and daddy love you, lots and tons and will be with you each step of the way.

Love you always,

Mom

June 6, 1994

Tomorrow we will be taking you to Cleveland clinic to have your heart defect repaired. The neighbor girls are over playing hospital with you and you are taking care of your doll which daddy drew a zipper boo-boo on.

We are all scared but we are going to be strong for you. You're a very strong little girl and you will be fine because I asked Jesus to send angels to watch over you and keep you safe. Mom and Dad will be with you too and we will never leave you. We LOVE you lots and tons.

Love,

Mommy

June 7, 1994

5a.m. We are driving to Cleveland Clinic and I am ready to tell daddy to turn around; but I know you need this to be healthy. I look back at you singing and smiling and I just ache inside. To us you are already our perfect little girl. You need this surgery, however, to make you even more perfect.

8a.m. We are at the clinic and they are prepping you for surgery. I'm trying really hard to keep it together and not fall apart until after you go in. They gave you a medication called Versiad (a mind altering medication so you will not remember). The medicine didn't seem to work. You cried because you wanted mommy to take you into the operating room. You don't want to go with the nurses. I put on scrubs and took you into the operating room and held you as we sang Jesus loves me until you fell asleep; it just about tore me up inside. Oh, Lord, keep her safe. Guide Dr. M.'s hands. With love and prayers, we leave you in his hands. I promise you that I will be there for you make sure you are in the best of hands. Remember that I love you and daddy does too!

Isaiah 66:13 *As a mother comforts her child, so will I comfort you.*

5p.m. Dr. M. told us you did super and the hole and valve were repaired. You are in PICU and we can go see you. You have tons of wires and tubes connected to you and you look so pale. We took Polaroid pictures so we could show family and friends who were waiting in the surgery waiting room. THANK GOD the surgery is over!!! We love you.

11:15p.m. Mom and Dad and Grandma went to get some sleep—I told them to wake me if you woke up.

June 8, 1994

12:05a.m. A knock at the door. You woke up. When we saw you the tube was out of your throat and you wanted a juice box. You were only allowed to have a teaspoon of liquid so even though hours ago you looked so weak, you stood up and demanded a juice box. Your dad and I could not hold you down. The alarms were flashing and beeping. Your heart rate was over 170. We finally got you calmed down and you immediately fell back asleep. Everyone at church is praying for you.

3:20p.m. We are settled down in your room. The PICU staff threw you out for being too rowdy. You rode in Mommy's lap in a wheel chair. We had to learn a whole new way of picking you up. For the next few months, you will need to sit down onto our arms instead of us picking you up under yours.

June 9, 1994

2:25a.m. Daddy went home around 10 for some sleep and to check on Knickers. They let me sleep in your room on a nice sleeper sofa. You just woke up screaming and it scared me to death. You had rolled over onto your belly in your sleep and put pressure on your chest. I laid next to you and you were out in a minute.

12:30p.m. June, Dr. M.'s nurse has been incredible! She has held our hand through every step so far. She took your I.V. out. It seems so unbelievable that we just took you for a wagon ride down the hall. You are doing so well. We are having to weigh your diapers to see how much liquid you put out and your liquid input is increased slowly. This is the hardest part for you. Daddy, Cindy and I have to sneak a pop in the hallway so you don't get mad. "I WANT MY JUICE BOX!!!"

June 10, 1994

You keep amazing us! You actually were feeling well enough to go out on the rooftop playground. You were all over the place. Dad even helped you go down the slide. It scared mommy but all is well. I hope you just did not overdo it.

June 11, 1994

11:00a.m. We are on our way home! We took some time getting pictures saying good-bye to your friends Lauren and Kevin. We also tracked down June. She was such an incredible help. We have such good family and friends who are taking good care of us.

GOD IS GOOD!!!

While spending time at Cleveland Clinic Children's Hospital, Dan and Julie talked with other parents and saw babies who suffered through much worse alone. They learned to say, "Only an ASD."

Megan is now fourteen, has no restrictions, and is in great health. She was the tallest player on her eighth grade basketball team this year and could run down almost anyone.

Dr. M. moved back to New Zealand and Akron Children's Hospital has opened a heart center where they perform surgery. Dan and Julie are both on the board of directors for HEALING HEARTS, which is currently coordinated by Katie Fleming, an incredible friend of families with CHD. Many lifelong friendships have been made there.

One of Dan and Julie's memories of HEALING HEARTS took place at the Thaxton's, friends of the family. On a hot summer day, after the food and annual romp through the woods, a small wading pool was brought from the garage. A garden hose pumped ice-cold water into it, and all the children enjoyed getting their feet wet.

That day, everyone knew they were blessed to be part of something larger and better than a 'support group'. They were in a great big 'no restrictions' club of love.

Dan and Julie thanked HEALING HEARTS for all they did to keep their child and others alive and well.

THE MURPHY FAMILY

Some families tend to have more health issues than others. Genetic factors may cause some of the problems. The Murphy family seemed to fit in this category.

Judy Murphy's grandparents and parents were born and raised in Tennessee where they worked as farmers. Her parents had three children while there, but later moved to Michigan, where Judy was born. The family then moved to Ohio where the parents worked at Chrysler. They had two sons born in Ohio.

Judy's father, George Edward Murphy, was a very hard working man who provided well for his large family. He worked at Chrysler in Twinsburg for thirty years. Although he was a very good father, he was not the best husband because he had affairs with women other than his wife. Everyone knew about the infidelity, but did not discuss it until after his death at age eighty-two.

George had been in good health, except for some stomach/ulcer problems, until age seventy-eight when he became diabetic and underwent heart surgery.

Although George was not very spiritual in his younger life, he believed in God. He drove his children to church every Sunday, but did not stay with them. However, two months before his death, he called Dora, his eldest daughter, to tell her he was saved and knew he would go to heaven when he died. During his last days, all of his children recognized the religious change in him. Although he had always told his children that he loved them when they were young, he now repeated this fact over and over.

Katherine Murphy, Judy's mother, passed away at age fifty-seven in 1979 from a blood clot in her lower arm that traveled to her heart. All of her life, she did not eat a healthy diet. She ate Southern fried, fatty foods every day. Katherine had diabetes and heart problems, and sometimes passed out from low or high blood sugars.

She knew Jesus as her Savior from a young age, and was a loving and hard working mother. Although she did not attend church regularly, she made sure her children did. Sunday found her at home preparing a large dinner.

During the week, she worked outside the home, mostly the night shift, so did not always get enough sleep. She took care of her home and children during the day.

The Murphy's first child, Dora, always lived a good Christian life. Her health problems included high cholesterol, high blood pressure, diabetes, fibromyalgia, clotted arteries, and heart problems. Although Dora never had a heart attack, she had eleven stents put in her arteries. At the present time, doctors will not perform open heart surgery on her because it is too much of a risk.

Dora retired from her job at age fifty-eight on disability, and firmly believes that she would not be alive today except for the Lord. The family held a big birthday party for Dora when she turned sixty years of age.

The Murphy's second child, a son, Eddie Evan, passed away when Judy was sixteen years old. He was married and had an eight month old son. Eddie had a lot of stomach/ulcer problems, and also had back surgery. After surgery, the doctor sewed him up and told the family he would only live about four hours. He explained that the ulcers ate up his back bone. Eddie died eight hours later. His condition today would be called cancer.

Judy prayed that Eddie's soul went to heaven, for he attended church with the rest of the children.

Kathy Diane Murphy, the third child, was always sickly. She was bed-ridden with rheumatic fever during the whole sixth grade of school. She had a rather bitter personality, even though she always received gifts from her parents that the other children did not. She even had her own cat.

Although Kathy went to church with the rest of the children, she never lived or acted like she knew God. She never talked to anyone about Jesus, sick or well. The day she died, she told Judy that she was ready to meet Jesus and her dead granddaughter in heaven.

Judy always felt close to Kathy and considered her to be her best friend until the day she died. Kathy passed away in 2001 at the age of fifty-one.

Kathy had worked at Chrysler and retired on disability at age forty-three. She had many health issues; diabetes, heart disease, open heart surgery, two or three stents, and congestive heart failure. At the time of her death, she was also on kidney dialysis.

Kathy had three daughters who are close to Judy to this very day. Judy and Kathy looked somewhat alike, and someone mistook Judy for Kathy at her brother's funeral. The person did not know that Kathy had passed on.

Judy Gail is the Murphy's fourth child and third daughter who was in good health all of her life until, at age forty, she found out that she had diabetes. At age forty-two, Judy had open heart surgery, and at age forty-five, surgery for her carotid artery on the right side of her neck. Judy does water exercise and takes medication for high cholesterol, high blood pressure, poor circulation, and fibromyalgia. However, at age fifty-three, she had a catheterization performed and three clogged arteries were discovered. Judy was thankful she did not have to have open heart surgery again. Instead, three stents were inserted.

Mother of two grown children, three step-daughters, grandmother of one blood grandson and ten step-grandchildren, Judy works forty or fifty hours a week, and cares for her disabled husband.

Judy lives one day at a time, is active in her church, and knows that when she dies, she will go to heaven.

Bob Cappie Murphy, age forty-eight, is the Murphy's fifth child. He has been in very good health all of his life, except he has had cataract surgery on his eyes. He does not have diabetes, but has some lower back pain and leg cramps.

For forty years of his life, he used drugs, and played hard rock music. He is divorced and has a harsh ex-wife.

Three years ago, he became active in his church and gave his life to Christ. Bob plays in the church orchestra and band. He uses his talents for the Lord, and his family is thankful for the positive change in his life.

The sixth child and third son, Donald David, died at age forty. Katherine was forty-two when he was born. Donnie weighed thirteen pounds, eleven and a half ounces. At birth, he was so big that the doctor pinched a nerve in his shoulder on delivery which caused his left arm to be small, and he also had palsy, which sometimes happens to large babies. This type of injury would never happen today because doctors perform a C-section instead of natural delivery.

Donnie had a rough life. His mother died when he was sixteen, which seemed to cause him angst towards life. His personality was like Kathy Diane's. Both of them felt like the world owed them everything.

Donnie never had much physical therapy to strengthen his small arm, so everyone felt sorry for him and babied and spoiled him before and after his mother's death. Afterwards, George married twice, and Donnie lived with two different step-mothers. Everyone else was grown and on their own.

The youngest son used drugs, mostly smoked pot. However, he never drank alcohol. He worked for five years in a factory in maintenance. At about age twenty-five, his health started deteriorating. He had diabetes, two heart attacks, congested heart failure, high cholesterol, high blood pressure, and large sores on his legs and feet.

Judy took care of Donnie the last two years of his life. She took him to the doctor and tried to get financial help for him. He had visiting nurse services, and meals on wheels. He did not receive his small disability checks until he was about thirty-two years old. Donnie never married, never had any children. He was always kind and loving toward Judy and told her "I love you" many times.

Two weeks before he died in the hospital, he told Judy that he could hardly wait to see Mommy in heaven. By his words, Judy was convinced he finally invited Jesus into his heart.

He expired during surgery while the doctors were putting an extra wire on his pacemaker. When Judy went to view his body in the operating room, the attending nurse asked her, "Are you Judy?

Judy replied, "Yes, I am."

The nurse said, "I want you to know that your name was the last word Donnie uttered."

Although Donnie had a sad life and an early death, Judy knows that there will be tears of happiness when they meet again in heaven.

A PHYSICIAN'S NONTRADITIONAL VIEWPOINT

Jessica was a physician who practiced emergency medicine and ultimately became the director of medical affairs for a group of urgent care centers. However, she began to see great deficiencies in the healing process of people, and controversy in certain types of surgery. She gradually acknowledged the fact that things seemed wrong, and started connecting to a higher source, namely God. She also believed that people can connect if they are simply respectful of each other's differences, and that we are all ONE as light beings living in a physical body.

Part of this conversion began one day when she had just returned from taking one daughter to soccer practice, helping the second daughter with her math problems, and listening to the third daughter complain about her less than perfect day.

Jessica began to feel overwhelmed because she stretched herself thinly and felt information overload at the same time. However, as she was watching the sliver of the moon through the kitchen window, she began to feel a sense of peace. Just then, the phone rang.

It was her dad calling to tell her that he had gone to the doctor and he was scheduled to have open heart surgery the next week. He added, "The doctor said that I either need to do this or I will die. Please don't worry. I just wanted you to know. I must call your brother now. Since I am tired, I won't keep you and we can talk at another time."

"But, wait," exclaimed Jessica, and asked, "Is Mom there?"

"Yes, here she is—later then?"

Her mother interjected, "Hello—so what else do you need to know?"

Jessica answered, "How did this come about? Did he have any symptoms? He did so well on the cruise last month."

"Well, we went for a checkup and he had a stress test which lead to a heart cath. And, no, he did not have any symptoms, but they say he is blocked and we have no choice. We have had a long day and are very tired."

Jessica replied, "Okay, Mom, I'll talk to you another time. I love you."

After the phone call, Jessica sat there stunned by the sudden turn of circumstances. She felt numb, and thought that she should just go to bed and think things through. She wanted to do the 'right thing' even though she was not sure what it was.

Her parents lived four hours away and she had three kids to take care of, so she could not just drop everything. Her life had taken on a lot of changes lately, and she no longer believed in surgery, but in the body healing without incisions.

This turning point occurred when she had lunch several years ago with a very famous heart surgeon. He told her that he came to the realization, after doing approximately 3,000 heart bypass surgeries, that healing does not occur with cutting. One of his patients whom he was unable to help given the friability of his arteries convinced him of this conclusion. He closed this particular patient without repair and simply told him to live life fully, without anger, hate, and so forth. The patient experienced a shift in energy and ten years later, he still felt good. The famous surgeon now does energy healing in Florida.

Jessica was moved by this powerful testimony and she researched it more by learning and experiencing all that she could in this field.

The next day was a typical busy day of kids' activities. Sometimes there is a pressure in keeping touch with the 21st century and all its demands. 'Quality time' is perhaps an illusion spent with the children you love.

Jessica decided not to go the post game soccer party, but her sweet daughter's phone call convinced her that she needed to change her plans.

Jessica felt resentful but had no other choice, so she quietly joined the crowd. The superficial conversations and triviality were in sharp contrast to the life and death situation that confronted her. She finally justified her somber mood by expressing that her dad was having a major surgery in just five days and she was trying to work through it. Jessica spoke to another physician at the party who offered a compassionate gesture to give a second opinion on the heart catheterization films. She arrived home exhausted, and fell asleep, but woke up in the middle of the night while thoughts kept flowing fast and distinct. She knew that it wasn't about films and tests, but about energy.

Jessica believed in what had been termed 'the field' which was a generic term for connecting to source or God and then knowing what it is that should or needs to be done. "I should not go the day of the surgery—I should stay home and work on keeping calm and connected so that Dad can survive the surgery. After all, energy healing has no distance and there are no boundaries. I know I will feel his pain and help him heal from a distance. When he does need me there in person, I will know." A peace overcame Jessica as she formed the plan. She called her parents and told them that she would be there but not in person until she felt that needed to change.

Jessica's parents understood because they knew their daughter would do what was best and also thought she should stay with her kids. Jessica believed that staying home was a better way to focus on 'holding the space' if anyone judged this decision. She was able to cope with it because of her firm belief.

The surgery would not have been Jessica's choice, but she could not sabotage her father's desires. He did not ask that she be present for the surgery. As a true healer or catalyst, Jessica let go of her personal feelings to allow that which is in divine order to take place. Letting go and trusting is all she had to do. She had taught many classes on how to create the portal to allow energy to flow. She knew she had to do this because it applied to her father, whom she loved dearly.

On the morning of the surgery, Jessica felt close to her father, even though she was two hundred miles away. Healing energy knows no distance. She tuned in to his feelings like a radio or TV channel, even more so than the phone calls. She found out that the surgery went well, even thought she knew that before the phone call, and he was doing fine in the intensive care unit.

That night, Jessica felt intractable pain and knew that she needed to go to her father. She called her mom in the morning to tell her that she was on her way.

After arriving at the hospital, her father seemed so fragile with the deep cuts inflicted on his body. She performed what some people call 'Reiki,' letting universal love flow through her hands. The grimace on his face disappeared while she sat by his side and administered the 'healing love'. Jessica was astounded by this experience, because she had never been taught anything similar as a physician. Drugs and protocols were what she practiced.

Jessica asked her dad, "How do you feel?"

He replied, "I feel relief from the pain, and am comfortable with the beautiful colors I see. Thank you, I feel better now that you are here."

Jessica knew that it wasn't her but she would be the tool for his healing to take place. She asked if she could get him anything to heal and help get him through this ordeal. She seemed to know the answer was that he needed protein to rebuild the torn tissue. The hospital provided sugar-free Jello and a salty broth that provided few nutrients, so Jessica went to the drug store that evening and bought him a protein shake that she thought would help him, again using her intuition to choose the right one. Right answers come if people allow them.

He gulped the shake and seemed to perk up. Jessica waited for divine guidance to trust that she would know when to return home to her family. She did not feel a sense of helplessness that she could tell others in the waiting room felt. There was no despair, but a realization on her part that she should try to teach others this way now that she had learned it herself.

The days dragged on, with many discussions of differences in belief, yet her family was looking to Jessica to help and relieve. This belief is really taught through being it and living it, not at all on a point of discussion. That peace and strength which Jessica felt was almost infectious to people around her, even though they did not really understand it. However, they derived a comfort which sparked their curiosity.

One day when everyone arrived expecting improvement, her dad said that he was saying good-bye because it was the 'end'. Jessica's mother and brother looked to her for an answer. Her reaction to her father's pale, diaphoretic, weak, and unhealthy looking condition was to be quiet and see things through divine eyes, not analytical or logical, which would require testing. She knew the answer would come to her when logic and thinking often fails in this type of circumstance.

Jessica suddenly knew that the pain pill he took in the morning was causing his reaction. Most people have no effect from Darvoset, but everyone is different. She told her family that they would know the answer whether it was the medicine or not in a few hours. It was her hunch that he would be okay.

However, these thoughts were interrupted by the surgeon who was very concerned and who ordered the usual series of tests immediately. Jessica instantly saw the insaneness of this 'fabulous' physician conducting these tests without connecting with her father. The physician relied on a knee reflex cerebral response that was customary and expected. She felt that she had been trained wrong, and questioned herself why she had been in this pathway at all. The tests, of course, showed no answers. Jessica proved to be right when, after four hours passed, and to everyone's amazement, her Dad returned to normal.

"How did you know? they questioned.

Jessica answered, "I just did."

It felt wonderful to have confirmation once again of this powerful process.

Jessica's father seemed to resonate and understand that people don't cross to the other side until their work is done here. Even if people live to be one hundred years old and are in a nursing home, they are here until their mission is complete. Father and daughter both knew at that moment that he had not completed his tasks on earth. He chose LIFE, and knew he would be fine. He must have felt that he was not ready to cross over yet.

After Jessica left for home, her father started to get a sense of purpose. He helped save his roommate's life by calling a nurse. His next roommate seemed to need a good ear for listening, and he was there for him. Since then, every day that comes his way is another day to BE the light and love for other people.

Jessica's father recovered on an amazing course and did not suffer one complication even though he was a diabetic. Science tells us that diabetics have trouble with wound healing, but that was not the case with him. He healed quickly and beautifully.

Jessica has shared this story to show that when people open their eyes to God as light beings in physical bodies, He is always there to lead us along and we simply need to ask to connect. "....and these and great things shall you do..." as stated in the Bible. She believes we were always meant to heal this way as Jesus taught us, and we can all be there for each other whenever we choose to serve. According to Jessica, each day is an amazing unfolding of events if one just stops to pay attention.

Printed in the United States
50443LVS00006B/202-264